Attention Deficit

Diagnosis and Treatment for Children and Adults With Add

(Discipline & Empower Kids With Attention Deficit Hyperactivity Disorder to Reach Success)

Irena Coleman

Published By **Simon Dough**

Irena Coleman

Attention Deficit: Diagnosis and Treatment for Children and Adults With Add (Discipline & Empower Kids With Attention Deficit Hyperactivity Disorder to Reach Success)

ISBN 978-1-998769-57-5

Legal & Disclaimer

Table of contents

Chapter 1: Add -- What It Is

It was first documented in the 17th century. However, the condition only became more common at the beginning of 19th century. Initially, it wasn't a diagnosed condition and was later given the name minimal brain dysfunction. The "ADDer", as I'll refer to them in this book is someone who can be inattentive and distractible, impulsive, hyperactive, disorganized, and impulsive. Others include being disorganized or hyperfocused, preservation (meaning that you are committed to completing something once you start it), and procrastinating.

ADD is referred to as a spectrum disease, meaning that it can affect a large or small range of human traits. These traits are a problem to ADDers. This is how it gained its name and reputation. An attention deficit can lead to ADDer children being unable to attend school. Or it can cause minor irritation. It is this range of disorders that psychiatrists use to diagnose and plan for treatment.

American Psychiatric Association conferred the name Attention Deficiency Disorder (ADD) on the condition in its "bible": Diagnostic Statistical Manual of Mental Disorders Fifth Edition. It's also known as the abbreviation DSM-5. DSM-5 also contained hyperactivity.

Being a family physician, I didn't find the term "attention deficit disorder" to be appropriate, especially for children. To tell a child they have "disorder" is to make it difficult for them and their parents to accept the diagnosis. Why? Because they are inclined to believe that something is wrong with them. There is nothing wrong with them, other than the fact that their brain functions slightly differently to their peers. You can see the relief on their faces when you tell them, using this language, that you have a processing issue and that your brain functions differently from other people's. It's a friendlier, more positive language than "attention disorder" and you can tell them that "you are broken." You have a disorder.

Dr. E. Hollowell has suggested changing the title to VAST. Hollowell is an authority in ADD. VAST stands for variable Attention Stimulation Trait. Notice that VAST stands for variable attention stimulation trait. Names with negative connotations are not included in VAST. Although I agree with the change, I expect the condition to continue to be known by its now infamous name--ADD.

In medicine, "diseases" and "illnesses are both terms used. A disease refers to a malfunctioning of the body. A sickness is an unhealthy condition in the body or mind that has been caused by the disease.

These names are not appropriate or helpful in explaining ADD. ADD does NOT qualify as a diagnosis or a disorder. I believe it's more appropriate to look at ADD as a condition, disorder, and not as a diagnosis or disease. In this book I'll refer to it in that way.

ADD can be seen in families as a condition that is inherited. It is impossible to determine which gene is responsible for ADD. Although there are multiple genetic markers for the condition that can be linked to it, no one has ever been able to identify a single gene. The disorder is multifactorial, involving multiple factors that affect brain function. "Condition" seems to be a more generalisation than "disease", or "illness".

I prefer to call the consequences of the condition "traits" and "behaviour pattern", rather than "symptoms", which is a negative word. Many of the ADD traits and behaviour patterns can be attributed to a lower level of executive functioning in the brain. Let's explore this more.

Executive Functioning

Depending on the book you are reading, the exact number of core functions the brain's executive functionality (EF), covers will vary. These EF process, along with cognitive controls (CC), are what control our behaviour. These processes are mainly found in the frontal lobes. ADD suffers have a significantly lower effectiveness. This is why ADD suffers need to be medicated more than non-ADD people. Another interesting fact is the difference in brain size between ADDers and healthy individuals.

The impact of a diminished EF function on ADDers can be varied and even very severe. This could affect almost all of their fundamental mental faculties. ADD can be very disruptive and destructive if the EF is not functioning properly. These resulting traits can often be controlled with proper treatment and monitoring by an ADDer.

Let's take a second to examine the most common ADD characteristics, as they are often seen in children and then in adults.

DSM Diagnostic Criteria for Childhood Addition

A child can have ADD if they exhibit the following behaviours or traits:

* Fidgeting

* Hyperactivity

* Distractibility

* Inability of waiting their turn

* Answering a question after the questioner is done speaking

* Difficulty following directions

* A lack of attention

* The act of switching from one activity into another

* Inability play quietly

* Talking in excess

* Intruding upon or interfering

* Not listening to what is said

* Losing things regularly

* Engaging with physically dangerous activities

ADD is a multifocal genetically inherited condition. This condition causes significant inattention and hyperfocus. The child ADDer is often unable and unwilling to be still during class. They are often referred to as "class clowns" and get into trouble for their bad behavior. Teachers often find that their performance is not as high as they expected. Their intelligence may not be as impressive as they would like, but their achievement isn't as high as they think.

DSM Diagnostic Criteria to Adult ADD

An adult suffering from ADD has a chronic disturbance that causes at least fifteen of these behaviours or traits to be present:

* Feelings demotivated

* No organization

* Procrastination

* Multiple simultaneous projects

* Blurting comments

* No stimulation required

* Boredom is a problem

* Distraction

* Creativity. Intuition. And Intelligence.

* Refusal to follow established channels

* Impatience

* Impulsivity

* Be Worried

* Feelings and sensations of insecurity

* Feelings can quickly change

* Restlessness

* Addictive behavior

* Lack of self-esteem

* Inaccurate self-observation

* Family history of ADD, mental illness, addictions

Adult ADDers might hide their condition by using self-engineered coping techniques or treating it. This masking can take place before or during diagnosis, and it is often not recognized by the ADDer. Adults with ADD initially delight in being able explain their poor performance and awkward behaviour. Most adult ADD symptoms are caused by the loss of certain aspects of their executive functioning. They lose the ability of managing themselves well. This inability is most noticeable in time management, planning and achieving the goals they have set. There are also many benefits to ADD in adults. There are many positive effects of ADD in adults, including creativity, impulsivity (impulsivity), inspiration, and the ability think creatively.

The traits of hyperfocus and intuition are also a part of ADD.

Types and Subtypes of ADD

Originally, ADD was believed to be composed of three subtypes. However other researchers have expanded that number to seven. These subtypes are useful for doctors to help them determine the best treatment. They also show a similar brain anatomy.

Three Types Of ADHD

1. ADHD predominantly hyperactive-impulsive presentation: least common

2. ADHD most often inattentive presentation

3. ADHD combined presentation: The most prevalent

DSM-5 Criteria to Diagnose ADHD

Add two more characteristics:

4. An ADDer will often avoid, dislike or be reluctant about tasks that require mental effort over a longer time.

5. The ADDer often misplaces essential items for tasks and activities.

Dr Amen's Seven Types of ADD

Dr Daniel Amen uses SPECT scanners to assess people with ADD. These scans are able to show specific patterns of blood flow in the brain. ADD decreases blood flow to affected areas. If a part becomes more active, blood flow increases. The scan will show a brighter area. Dr Amen has been able to classify seven kinds of ADD based on this fact. It is important to note that not all researchers can interpret these scans correctly and consistently. This attitude seems to be a little too cautious, even after over thirty years.

Here are the seven categories of ADD that Dr Amen based on SPECT scans.

1. Classic ADD--symptoms include inattention and distractibility, hyperactivity, disorganisation, impulsivity,

and normal brain activity at rest. Concentrated tasks show decreased brain activity.

Dopamine deficiencies with reduced blood supply to the cerebellum, prefrontal cortex, and basal-ganglia.

Treatment: Adderall and Vyvanse stimulants.

2. Inattentive ADD - A short attention span, distractibility (maybe daydreaming), and disorganised procrastination.

Causes: Low activity of the prefrontal cortex.

Treatment: Adderall or Vyvanse stimulants.

3. Over-Focused ADD - The core symptoms of classic ADD are difficulty shifting attention, thought and task; getting stuck on negative thoughts; and inflexibility.

Inflexibility means a failure to see alternatives.

Causes: Dopamine and Serotonin Deficits; Overactive Anterior Cingulate Gyrus

Treatments: Antidepressants, amino acids, and Neurofeedback

4. Temporal Lobe ADD - Core symptoms of classical ADD. Learning, memory and behavioural problems. Anger, aggression and paranoia.

Causes: Abnormalities of the temporal lobe, decreased function in prefrontal cortex

Treatment: GABA (gamma aminobutyric acids) amino acid; anticonvulsants used to treat mood stability

5. Limbic ADD - Core classic ADD; along with chronic low-level sadness and moodiness; low energy levels;

helplessness; guilt with chronic low self esteem

Causes: An overactive limbic region of the brain (mood management); reduced activity in prefrontal cortex

Treatment: amino acids, atypical antidepressants like Wellbutrin.

6. Ring of Fire AD--sensitivity to light touch and noise; mean, nasty and unpredictable behaviour; fast speaking; anxiety and fearfulness

Causes: A hyperactive ring around the brain.

Treatment: Anticonvulsants, elimination diet, amino acid, anticonvulsants, blood pressure medication, and anticonvulsants to calm hyperactivity.

7. Anxious ADD -core symptoms of classical ADD. Anxiety with generalised stress and fear that you will be judged.

Causes: Basal ganglia hyperactive (opposite most types ADD)

Treatment: Relaxation and not the use of stimulants; neurofeedback is used to reduce symptoms of anxiety

My Personal Diagnosis

Dr Amen did not have a classification for me when I was diagnosed with ADD at 55. I was diagnosed with ADD by my pediatric psychiatrist. Many experts advise adults to consult a child psychiatrist. This is because they are often able to treat adults with ADD.

Dr Amen has identified seven types of ADD. Although I've never been to a SPECT, it is certain that I suffer from the fifth, limbic ADD. The limbic systems is found deep within the brain, on the left and right sides of the thalamus. It is below the medial temporal lobes of cerebrum. The limbic effect can cause low self-esteem, sadness and helplessness, along with a lack energy, moodiness and depression. My symptoms are typical of limbic ADD.

My entire life I have been dysthymic. Five years ago, my GP diagnosed me with ADD. What I saw in my life was that I was quickly embarrassed, had low self esteem and struggled with relationships.

I was initially diagnosed with ADD. It helped me understand my depressive symptoms and my education issues. My ADD diagnosis helped to explain my delay in completing medical school. I was only able do so at the age of 28. The decade between the end of high school and the start of medical school was the period I needed in order to mature enough for higher education. I realized this when I received my ADD diagnoses at 55.

ADD and Emotional Sensoriivity

The most cutting-edge research into ADD shows that people with ADD have an extreme sensitivity to what others think and say about them. Dr William Dobson reports that people with ADD are sensitive to emotions, particularly feelings of shame and guilt that can be exacerbated when they receive rejection. This rejection sensitive dysphoria has been described by Dobson as RSD. The Greek word dysphoria, which literally means "hard-to-bear", is what the term "dysphoria", comes from. This RSD is very evident when someone with ADD perceives reject.

RSD sufferers can be easily upset by criticisms of others, even though it isn't true. Adults and teenagers with ADD can be more sensitive than others to rejection. This condition requires the person to work extremely hard so others will admire and like them. You might withdraw from social activities and develop an phobia. Social phobia refers to a severe fear of being embarrassed when speaking in public. RSD has been shown in studies to impact the relationships of ADDers with their families, friends and romantic partners.

The following are signs of rejection sensitive disorder (RSD).

* Being easily embarrassed

* Anger or emotional outbursts after being hurt or rejected.

* Setting very high standards, which they often fail to meet.

* Feeling low self-esteem

* Always feeling anxious, especially when you are in social settings

* Having difficulties with relationships

* Avoiding social situations.

* Feeling like an failure because they haven't lived up to their own expectations

* Sometimes people think about hurting themselves.

The above list of symptoms could indicate that someone with RSD has a variety of other mental disorders. This is an example:

* Bipolar disorder

* Borderline personality disorder

* Post-traumatic stress Disorder (PTSD).

* Obsessive-compulsive disorder (OCD)

* Depression

* Social phobia

In my teens, rejection sensitive disorder was a very visible part of me. It caused anxiety and embarrassment. I struggled with the way people perceived me. I also felt like an unjustified failure.

RSD is a completely new and different aspect of ADD. It is only now that some of my feelings are clear. This is the reason why I was unable to speak openly about this aspect of ADD until recently. Sandra, my spouse, noted that I was more cooperative when she asked me to do chores around the home. This is the flip side of RSD: RE.

The Other Side: Recognition Responsive Eugenia (RRE).

When someone with ADD receives praise and encouragement in their activities, they experience a very different emotional response. The opposite of RSD is experienced by someone with ADD when they are given praise and support. It's a dramatic emotional reaction that can lead to recognition responsive euphoria, or RRE.

Personally, I know how it feels to feel euphoric when someone compliments me on something I did. In my case, the patients who wrote me a thank you note when I was working in an ER are a rare and special example of how much I appreciate it. Any indirect compliments from my colleagues that informed me of how well I managed a particular case were very pleasant to me. After a long night in the ER, I will remember a simple compliment from a senior staff nurse. She stated, "We did all do well", but she also said, "I still have to understand how you Dr Norman are able keep up with the demands."

Even now, while I was waiting in a line to enter the grocery store, a man two ahead of me said, "Hi, Dr Norman". I answered in a vague way. His response was vague. The lady in the middle of us said, "And mine two." Both admitted that all of these babies were now adults, with their own children. This recognition made it great for me. I regret that I did not recognize them.

In the next chapter we will look at how ADD develops, from intrauterine to adulthood.

Chapter 2: Add Development And Causes

Multiple causes can lead to ADD and are not well understood. It could be caused by head trauma as a growing child or intrauterine. It is well known that the condition can be caused by any one of these. ADD can still be passed down from one generation to the next.

Some experts consider preterm births and low birth weight to significant causes. Others suggest that it is caused by a loss in maternal-baby bonding in the baby's first year. Others believe unremembered injuries to the head can trigger the condition. Some even argue that the situation is an echo of hunter-gatherer tribal life, hundreds of thousand years ago. They claim that ADD sufferers are descendants of tribe hunters.

Development of ADD

Currently, ADD experts disagree about the various environmental and developmental aspects of this disease.

There is no doubt that ADD is a major cause. But it is not damage to one or an abnormality in any particular gene. Often when dealing with an adult with ADD after treatment has been successful, the parent will return to their doctor suddenly with one of their children. Usually, they bring along a son whom they believe may also have ADD. Also, the converse is very common. A teacher may say that a child has ADD. When the child is evaluated, the parent or both parents confess to similar behavior. Popular genetics testing does not prove that someone is in fact a carrier of the suspected genes.

This chapter continues chronologically and discusses many of the contributing factors and causes that could lead to ADD.

Intrauterine

Many researchers believe that ADD begins in the uterus during the baby's development. A few people mention the fact some babies can get so excited in the womb, they can kick their mothers, sometimes even causing her to have a broken rib. They can be so active it's like trying to keep hold of a salmon. They are extremely hyperactive and appear to have this problem since birth. This idea has been proposed only recently. Due to the circumstances, it is not possible and medically ethical to investigate it in order to determine if it could be harmful to a fetus.

Birth

Prematurity is a main factor in many of the problems that can arise from life. Low birth weight could also be an issue. Extended labour could cause problems.

Other factors that could contribute include temporary hypoxia (lack or oxygen) and physical trauma such as a forceps delivery.

Baby

Experts in ADD feel that the illness can be caused by problems between mother and child that happen around one-year old. In Dr Gabor Mate's book Scattered Minds Dr Mate suggests that babies can experience a profound affect on their mothers if they lose contact with them. This loss of connection must be immediate, severe, and sustained. The baby may feel that they are isolated, and so they cut off any normal bonding smiles. The precipitating factor can be loss of direct contact and subsequent development ADD.

Other causes may be due to many factors. For example, the mother might be required to go work because of her environment. When the mother is being held in jail for a crime and cannot have contact with her baby, it's called social stress. Another possible cause is severe postpartum depression, in which the mother is sent to hospital and then separated from her baby.

It is possible that this was the case for children born to mothers separated during World War Two. Evidence suggests that such babies are brought up in large numbers with little or no supervision from their caregivers. This leads to severe mental problems in these babies, and ADD is often a later diagnosis.

In my situation, it seems that there might have been a separation from my mother. Unfortunately, this is not something I can confirm. I do recall her telling me that my father had hired a housekeeper/nanny who was highly recommended to her, shortly after I was born. She also said that she refused to allow the lady to get involved with her. The nanny drove me out of the house in my pram. I cried for days. I eventually accepted the situation and settled down. I never understood the reasons for my mother's housekeeper coming to her aid. I now wonder if my mother (an elderly primigravida, or first pregnancy) at 35, suffered from postpartum depressive symptoms. Aside from the fact that I was eight-weeks premature and very low in birth weight, there is also that in my case.

Preschool

It has only been recently that we have realized the importance of this stage in development for a child's growth. Preschool covers children from 2 to 5. A lack of interaction with other young children, and learning how to play is often the issue at this stage. Good socialization starts with interactions with other children. The child will become self-centered if they are not able to make contact with their peers. Children often form fictitious friendships during this period. They can share their thoughts and concerns with them. This is the period that is believed to mark the beginning of self-talk in the future, which can have a significant controlling influence on a person's development.

I was shocked when, as a young medical student in my first year, I discovered that the most significant learning and development occur in the first years of our lives. It is only when you look at this that you realize how the child learns to recognize their mother, siblings and pets. They also begin to speak slowly during this year. The child is also learning to run and walk, and hopefully climbing safely. A child suffering from ADD may not feel threatened or afraid of heights.

Primary School

ADD can manifest in primary school when a child reaches the age of five to eleven. The child will often be hyperactive and unable sit still. Teachers have a hard time getting the affected child down. As I mentioned earlier, the class sees the pupil as the class clown. However, if you read the literature, it is clear that some of our most successful comedians had ADD. Other children may seem very quiet and scattered out. This is often true for girls with ADD. It is because of this that some young women who had ADD were not recognized when they were given the diagnosis to explain their poor school performance.

This is usually where the attentive teacher states in the report card the child with ADD that they could be doing better. Children with ADD can find the teacher a tremendous support. They can alert parents to their suspicions of ADD.

However, their greatest benefit is for the pupil. An educator can make a huge difference in the lives of children with ADD by offering encouragement and alternative stimulation. An author who had ADD himself mentioned a teacher, a professor, and a relative when he was referring to a referenced textbook on ADD. They had all helped him deal with and profit from his ADD. With the support of their parents, the child often receives the best treatment and can improve his grades significantly. It is important to remember that many of these children are trying very hard and making silly and stupid mistakes. It is not acceptable to shout at these children and tell them that they need to be more focused. Concentration is not the issue. They can focus, but their inattention and desire to be perfect is more of a problem.

Primary school is when we begin to see the child develop interpersonal skills.

Often in an ADDer these skills are not present. An ADD person is often a loner who has few or no friends. They are often shunned by their peers because of their behavior. This could be because the ADDer interrupts other students constantly or tries to take over.

High School

High school is where ADDers can have problems with many of the technical aspects. ADD is a disorder that makes it difficult to learn math, science, reading, reciting, and arithmetic. Some children struggle with numbers and mathematics, while others have terrible fears of reading aloud to classmates. Without parental involvement, they are often late on most of their assignments. You can find out if your child has ADD by asking the parent how long they need to complete their homework. It's not normal for homework to take too long and shouldn't take all night. However, if a child's homework takes longer than expected, it could indicate that they may have ADD.

There should be a treatment plan, as well as all the assistance needed at home, to help the ADDer get to school on time. To learn punctuality and to be on time for school. Children affected by this condition need constant reminders about appointments. Time management is the most difficult problem to treat. You can use appropriate aids, such a notepad and a pen or even a smartphone to help you manage your symptoms. It's helpful.

Recreation is an often overlooked aspect of teenage living. There are many types of recreation, but for ADDers, they must be involved in some kind of hard-working sport to burn off some of their extra energy. A second thing that I feel is crucial and often overlooked, is to encourage ADD children in their youth organizations, such as Boy Scouts or churches. Socialization among teenagers through clubs, teams, and organizations is one the most cost-effective, effective, and efficient ways to improve social skills. The ADDer needs to be taught swimming skills and should also be taught basic first aid. Participating in community activities with the ADDer is a good option if they have the time. It allows them to interact with adults and with strangers.

A mentor, someone who shows the ADD child what to do and encourages them, can be a huge help. Mentors can come from any source, including their teacher, a sibling and even a classmate. A tutor can be a mentor for children with ADD. They will help them with math, science, geography and history. Often, the tutor can be an older student and is rewarded for helping the ADDer.

Hopefully by the time the ADDer reaches high school, they are able to have some ideas about a career path. Encourage them to take on tasks that are appropriate for their ADD. A good example of this is to tell ADD kids not to do monotonous jobs. They will find it boring and tedious, which can be counterproductive to what ADD is strong at. ADDers should be encouraged and supported to pursue their interests in arts, music, dramas, science, mathematics, business, or any other related fields.

Post-School Training - Trades, College or University

The ADDer may desire to have a job after secondary school. I recommend that they take driving lessons prior to that. From my experience as a GP and having seen unplanned pregnancies in patients, I recommend that the ADDer get advice about sexuality.

College is where you start your adult life. Colleges are not for students. This is especially true for ADDers who take university courses. The orientation is provided by universities and colleges to help students get started in their courses. Students then take responsibility for their actions. They are responsible for submitting assignments on-time and presenting for examinations. The students decide if they want to attend lectures. However, they will often be required to keep an attendance record in order to receive hands-on training. The university does not care much about a student's attendance. But, I know from personal experience that they will assist students in the event of a serious incident.

Even though ADDers are just starting out in the workforce, students at colleges and universities should be responsible for their own lives, like all their peers. Parents and the ADDer may seek out additional support at the institution because of their condition. Parents who notice ADDer's behavior is different than their peers should inform any educators or employers about it. Ask if the educator or employer would be willing and able to provide any assistance. The parents need to intervene if the ADDer begins working but is then fired. If the reason for dismissal is because of poor time management, then the ADDer must take every step to remedy the problem. All ADD students who are enrolled in college or university have to follow the same rules. Parents should confirm that the ADDer is present at school and submit all assignments on time. The ADDer must find out if their university or college allows them to be mentored so that they can stay on the right track.

Community college is often the place where trades can be taught. It typically involves some sort of sandwich course. This means that six months are spent at work (apprenticeship), followed by six months at college. This is a reminder of what needs to be done and the best way to do it: an employer can often be a huge help with advising and assisting ADD students as they attend college. To make this happen, the ADDer must talk to their college or employer. They should ask for specific guidance and support.

Future Career

Adults with ADD have a lot of difficulty choosing a future career. The career choice should be tailored to the individual's abilities and interests. The most common mistake is to try to put a square peg in a circle hole. A person's ADD traits must be matched with their future career. Although I am an accountant, I would not encourage a hyperactive, impulsive ADDer into law or accounting.

But it is well-known that ADD can make some courtroom lawyers very successful. The second aspect of this is that ADDers need to enjoy the career they are pursuing.

The two most important decisions a person can make in life are, as I see it. The first is finding a partner who is supportive and suitable. The second is finding a job that is suitable for you. Let's start by discussing the importance of choosing appropriate work. A person with ADD should choose a job that matches their interests, aptitudes, and capabilities, while still allowing them the opportunity to succeed and enjoy life.

I was able to see Dr Hallowell in a YouTube session. When an ADDer is contemplating their future career, he suggested that they make a list with three headings: What are you good at, What are you interested in, And what would you be paid. If you are looking for employment opportunities in the future, it is worth looking into how these three categories interact. If an adult with ADD is happy and stimulated, a career change may not be necessary. However, if the individual is unhappy or unable to do their current job, it might give them a better idea of what kind of career they might like.

I could go on for hours about recommending careers, but I will stop with Sir Richard Branson, his book called Screw It. Let's Make It: Lessons From Life.

Let's examine the importance of choosing the right partner to be your life partner. It is essential to have a wonderful life with the right partner for someone suffering from ADD. Your partner must be open to accepting you as you present and encouraging you to develop. My wife keeps reminding me of my accomplishments, even now.

Social

Social category is responsible for happiness, wealth, and health. The ADDer has to take care of himself, just like everyone else. They must eat well, adequately, and properly. People with ADD must also exercise regularly. You should make it more challenging for them to exercise when they're younger. They should, just like everyone else try to manage their weight. The ADDer should appreciate the fruits of hard work as well as their wealth. They should be aware and willing to help those less fortunate in society.

Happiness is found in all areas of life, including the personal, social and spiritual. Spiritual happiness can be described as taking care of your spirit in whatever way suits you. One of the most common would be religion. Other options include regular contact outdoors and with nature. For me, human happiness means having an interest which continually challenges you. You should be passionate about it, and you should learn how to collaborate with people with similar interests. This could include being a part of a service club such as Rotary or participating in athletic training.

I am grateful that I joined Brandon Rotary Club. I am an active honorary club member. I was also fascinated by the geography of Southwest Manitoba. Brandon University's professor of geography made me friends and educated me extensively about the geography south of Manitoba. Another friend owns a plane, and I fly regularly with him. Many years ago, I flew to Oshkosh in order to attend the Experimental Aircraft Association weeklong Fly-In meeting.

Personal happiness is my number one priority for a fulfilling life. Your family, friends and coworkers are the most important. Your partner, your spouse, your lover, and the person who is most important in your life, are all essential members of this group. As important and challenging as picking the right career is choosing a partner.

Now that we have taken a larger picture of ADD development, let's take a look at how it is diagnosed.

Chapter 3: Assessment And Diagnosis

It is not possible to diagnose this condition with one test. A team of physicians should examine the ADDer. This is the only way to diagnose the condition. The team should include a psychiatrist, or a competently trained doctor. They interview the person to learn more about their motivations, future goals, and past behavior. They obtain confirming statements from the ADDer's parents, spouse, children, siblings, grandparents, and, if possible, their teachers and close friends. You can also complete several assessment questionnaires like the World Health Organization's Adult ADHD Self-Reporting Scale. The ASRS can often confirm the diagnosis. It is possible to create a differential diagnoses based on all the background information. The examiner will then be able to obtain a complete picture and diagnose the patient.

Many psychiatric illnesses can mimic ADD. And even some conditions can be present alongside ADD. This possible diagnostic ambiguity can be explained by the fact that ADD often has comorbidities. These are conditions where two chronic conditions or diseases are present in a patient. This includes depression. However, there are many other conditions that can be co-occurred with ADD, including anxiety. You might also be interested in:

* OCD obsessive-compulsive disorder

* ODD oppositional defiant disorder

* ASPD antisocial temperament disorder

* SPD sensory processing disorder

* CD conduct disorder

* Post-traumatic stress disorder (PTSD)

Most likely, the person was sent for multiple blood tests to determine if they have thyroid disease, anaemia or diabetes mellitus.

Other than depression and comorbidities there are many other medical conditions and psychiatric diagnoses you should avoid. These may include multiple sclerosis, a space-occupying tumour (brain cancer), schizophrenia, and any other mental or physical condition. A person assessing an adult might need to go through all of their documents at home. They will need copies of their school report cards with comments from teachers. Coworkers, family, friends, and employers may also be needed. A criminal record, any history of drug abuse, driving records, and evidence of the person's marital status are all vital. The psychiatrist reviews the findings with the person, and then a final diagnosis is made. Let's now discuss the psychiatrist's role.

Psychiatrist

Consultation with a psychiatrist or other qualified doctor is necessary to determine if an individual has ADD. They need to evaluate the personality and interests of potential ADDers, as well as what triggers anger or makes them laugh. The team needs to have detailed information about each person. The person's prior medical history. This includes whether or not they have been diagnosed with any diseases. What is the current state of their health?

The psychiatrist must rule out any other possible diagnoses. ADD patients should be aware of depression as it is the most important comorbidity. These comorbidities often mask or even become the primary illness, i.e. post-traumatic stress disorder (PTSD), multiple sclerosis, MS.

The most crucial aspect of a diagnosis can often be found in the history that the ADDer provides about their problems and how they affect them. You could use simple examples like the state of their workspace. They can also be very clear about their time management, money management, and how they behave. It is their ability or inability, to concentrate and think clearly about a task until it is finished. They are asked to observe for procrastination. Sometimes, the person will benefit from answering the question "Why do you come here?" What did their employer send? Or were they referred to by the courts? Is it just curiosity? Is it possible that one of their children has been diagnosed with ADD recently and the parents feel the child is just like them?

Psychologist

Psychologists may also be a useful member of the assessment group. A psychologist can often provide valuable additional information through psychological testing. A full psychological assessment would be beneficial to the person being tested. The psychologist would administer multiple psychological tests. An examination may include a TOVA test to determine the variables of attention. The psychologist will order multiple investigations. Some of the more thorough ones are meant to pinpoint someone suffering from ADD. Other procedures that may be requested could include quantitative electroencephalography (qEEG). The brain mapping procedure, or quantitative electroencephalography (qEEG), measures the brain's electrical activity. A computerisedtomogram (CT), scan will be able to rule any gross anatomical cerebral issues. Finally, functional magnetic resonance image scanning (fMRI), also measures cerebral bloodflow and provides a measure of neuronal activity.

SPECT Scans

We talked about Dr Amen and his pioneering use of SPECT scanners to identify seven types ADD based primarily on blood flow patterns. I'll talk a little more about his SPECT findings. SPECT-Single-photon emission computed tomography--scanning has been used successfully to map out all the functional parts of the human mind. These types of scans are used to show which areas of the brain function normally and which are inactive or overactive. The SPECT scans show areas of the brain that are active or asleep, and can also reveal if medications have influenced the brain. This type is useful for determining which form of ADD a person might have. After many years, some authorities continue to question the accuracy of these scans.

My Diagnosis

There are several points of concern in the case of my diagnosis. As previously mentioned, I was delivered eight weeks early and born with low birthweight to my mother, an elderly primigravida. She was also my first and only child. My mother had to "rest" so I was taken from my mother when I was a child. It is possible that she was suffering from postpartum Depression.

Timmy, my imaginary companion, was there for me throughout childhood. I talked to him often and he accompanied me. Gem, a Springer Spaniel and my other companion, was Gem. My teachers told me at primary school that I could do better by putting in more effort. My inappropriate behaviour was often a problem. When the headmaster entered and told the class that King George VI had been killed, I laughed. (I should also mention that I was born and raised in Scotland. I moved to Canada once I was a teenager.

At secondary school, it became clear that I was a slow reader and poor reader, with very little understanding. I was able to do reasonably well in the subjects that I enjoyed. It was still difficult if the subject required me to read and memorize a lot, such as English language or history.

It was at this moment that I realized one of the most difficult problems I faced as teenager. My birthday is 26 March. My father decided arbitrarily that I must have written a letter of thanks to all who sent me Christmas presents prior to my birthday. These letters must be written in cursive. One occasion, he became very angry at me because I was wasting good writing papers. I wasn't able to understand why I was "so stupid", neither did he. Unfortunately, the answer was revealed many years later than he had expected. Only one thing he accomplished was that I hate writing on paper, especially letters. I enjoy typing letters or notes on a laptop with a spellchecker (what I'm using to create this book). I recall being criticized by one stenographer about my grammar and spelling. She quickly corrected me and said that she was a GP.

High school: Impulsivity was the dominant trait. Two of these incidents merit comment. I was told by my classroom teacher that she wanted me in another class. I found out the number of the classroom and began to investigate further. It was a class full of girls learning how to type. (Unfortunately I was too slow for my age, and hadn't found out anything about girls! I turned down the class immediately, and I regret it ever since. I know that I would have improved my English comprehension and reading speed if it had been taken. Maybe I would be typing the book instead of typing it into a Microsoft Word computer with Dragon Dictate. Another hilarious incident occurred. I was deep in thought as I sat at the back a class on engineering and mechanics when I was asked by my teacher to throw up some chalk. I did what the teacher asked, throwing it in my hands. It ended up smashing on the blackboard. The teacher responded nonchalantly by saying, "Next time you lob it underhanded."

Let's now look at the five years that passed before I was diagnosed with adult ADD. It would have been around 50. I was on depression treatment at that time and maintained that I was not suffering from depression. I acknowledged that I was a dysthymic (a sort of glass-isn't-half-full state of being). I was referred to two psychiatrists. The first one was a local one, and the second one was one I found in Winnipeg. Both psychiatrists diagnosed me with depressive symptoms. Five years later when I was diagnosed with ADD and given a diagnosis, neither of these psychiatrists knew much about A.D.D.

Child psychiatrist was the person who first diagnosed me with ADD. I went through a number of psychological tests. I also had an interview. The psychiatrist was certain that I suffered from ADD. After that, I was referred by a Winnipeg psychologist who conducted a series of psychological tests as well as ordered a Test of the Variables in Attention. It measures the speed at which you respond to stimuli and the response time of your computer. She claimed that I was only patient who fell asleep during the TOVA test. I disagreed and didn't believe that I had been asleep. To be fair, it wasn't 8:30 am and I had driven over 200 kms to get there. It was also before 5:00. Once again, she confirmed the diagnosis and said that I had suffered from ADD my whole life.

You must realize that the last five years were not my choice. My general practitioner, a friend and colleague, as well as two psychiatrists, had treated me for depression. They made me take Prozac (the new miracle drug), which I did for a time, but it was not of any real benefit.

After the confirmation of my ADD diagnosis, Ritalin was given to me. My wife believes that Ritalin helped me be more efficient with my daily life. My wife is certain that Ritalin made me more flexible, responsive, efficient, and consistent in completing routine household tasks. I felt as though I was going out to get a Scotch (whisky) every morning. I did not feel drunk, but I felt like I was floating in a fog. It was a way of being that I didn't like. I wrongly stopped using the drug. This led to me not being able to take any medication for the limbic form of ADD for the next 15 years. Wellbutrin, the medication I use for it. It took me 15 year to finally accept my ADD diagnosis.

Chapter 4: Assimilation

Once a person has been diagnosed, it is possible to begin refocusing. This refocusing helps ADDers to learn and understand many aspects. This is a time when the ADDer can gather all of their issues and seperate them into two types: those they perceive are effective (good), or those they view as deficient (bad). To aid me in understanding my ADD, I came up with the idea of affective (AS), which can be caused or exacerbated by my ADD. I then subdivided them in to either an effective state (ES; advantageous) and a defective state (DS: disadvantageous). Each ADDer must determine if there is an affective state. They will then need to determine if the effect has an ES/DS. (We'll be discussing three of my deficient states, chapters 7 through 9, in Chapters 7 to 9).

It is a time to recognize the benefits and disadvantages the condition has bestowed on the ADDer. First, you need to know what ADD is. I will cover four of these more common traits in chapter 6.

It is important to remember that ADD has both negatives and positives. The pros and con of ADD are most evident in the adult, and especially in those who have suffered for years with no symptoms. This complex process involves assimilating all the knowledge about ADD, and especially adult ADD. This chapter will focus on the process of assimilation.

Adult ADD, if not diagnosed early on, could lead to a variety of issues. Some issues may be very severe. For example, they could lose their university job or get fired. Other problems could include poor timekeeping, being late for work and a lack of discipline. The ADDer may also have other issues, such as an addiction to alcohol or drugs, sex, hoarding and accumulating unnecessary things, a lack in financial control, or binge eating or shopping. These are just some of the possible problems.

Diagnosis: Response

Consider the effects of this information on the ADDer when you get the diagnosis. For many, the relief that ADDers feel when they learn of their diagnosis is significant, particularly for those who are not yet diagnosed. Why? Because it provides an explanation to the ADDer, and sometimes even justification for their behavior. It also gives the ADDer a means to address and even manage the difficulties that it has caused. We hope that one day, the adult will be able to accept the diagnosis and use the new information for their clinical benefit.

However, some people with ADD cannot benefit from this knowledge. Some individuals with ADD must change their behaviors and how they present to be treated. Some refuse to change. Some people refuse to change because they feel it is unfair to be ridiculed and criticised for their current behavior. This is often seen in people who have a job that is not very fulfilling but who are afraid to inform their employers about their diagnosis.

It is also important to determine if ADD is a positive or negative condition. For some adults, it is possible to review their lives to see how ADD has benefited. Other adults may be able to review their lives to see if ADD has hindered them. Let me show you some examples.

There are many advantages to ADD, particularly for certain professions. These include positions such as a courtroom lawyer or fireman, a police officer or fireman, an ambulance crew member, or even an ER physician. These professions require individuals who are able think on their own, quickly come up with a conclusion and deal with what has happened. A diagnosis of ADD may help an adult ambulance driver to understand how the hyperfocus traits and impulsivity associated with ADD have helped them in their career.

It is also true for the reverse. I'll give you a more detailed explanation. My medical school experience included a new, exciting course called medical sociology. Many of our more senior professors opposed the addition to our curriculum of this course. In my case, the course was unbelievably useful in explaining many of these issues to sufferers. I am a busy GP who also works as an ER doctor. In this class, there was much discussion about addictions. We discussed whether smoking, alcohol, or drugs were the reasons. This question was again raised in psychiatry many years later. However, no one could agree on how to fix it.

We know today that ADD sufferers can use drugs and alcohol as a form treatment.

The adult population is often affected by the same addictions as the children. This observation raises the question of whether these conditions might have a genetic basis. It's now common knowledge that addictions can be caused by ADD in adults. These addicts find relief from their ADD symptoms via smoking, drinking alcohol, and taking drugs. These addictions can have far more severe consequences. It becomes clear that adult ADD is a condition that is prevalent in many people, but very visible in a large number of prisoners in our prisons. If someone with ADD develops addictions and ends up in jail, it is possible that ADD played a major role in their lives.

Those who spend their entire adult lives acting "oddly", with few or no friends, and engaging in illegal activities often are deemed to have ADD. When they learn that the reason for their stupid behavior is medical, they often hide it from their loved ones, friends, and coworkers. This information, which they get from an ADD diagnosis, is a dual-edged sword. While it may explain some of their symptoms and expose them to having to accept the diagnosis, it also presents a challenge. Imagine the ADDer who works in a low-paying job and is subject to ridicule and even abuse from their superiors. They are forced to live their lives hiding their ADD symptoms.

ADD sufferers don't all need to be Winston Churchill, Tony Phelps and Richard Branson. Many are simply lonely employees doing low-wage jobs just to make ends work. A person with ADD may have a criminal record. This is usually due to some type of addiction which encourages them in other illegal activities, such as assault or stealing. Their bad behavior often leads to them being brought to the attention police. Another example is a teenage girl who becomes a single parent and has one or two kids. This is due to impulsivity with ADD. These are examples I believe of the affected branch that I associate ADD with.

If a person has been diagnosed with ADD they have the right to decide if their condition is helpful (effective or ES), or obstructive. Once they make that decision, the next step for them is to learn everything about the condition. They will then need to use that information as a guideline to help them get past as many of the negative effects as possible, and then they can hopefully enjoy the rest.

This is a complex process that requires a lot of effort to integrate all of the information regarding ADD and especially undiagnosed adult ADD. This process can also be broken down into three parts: psyche (personal), and people.

Psyche

Psyche, or the brain's ability absorb, assimilate and interpret the new information when a person is diagnosed with ADD. The ADDer might not be aware of this, but it is still taking place. At a subliminal level, the ADDer needs to revise many subliminal processing to accommodate the new diagnosis. This is analogous to the development processes that are unobserved in a one year-old baby. It is hoped that adult ADDers will rise to the occasion.

I felt relieved to learn that I was not suffering from depression after I was diagnosed. It was because I didn't enjoy the way Ritalin made my feel that I decided to stop taking it. And, since I was a doctor, I believed I was right in making that decision. There is a saying in the professions--accountants should not look after their own financial affairs; lawyers should not be their legal counsellors, and doctors should not treat themselves, their family, or friends. To be fair, my type of ADD has been treated for approximately ten year.

Personal

It is likely that the most important aspect in adult ADDers' assimilation is their "personal" aspect. It is the individual acceptance and understanding that ADD is a condition. The ADDer should accept their new diagnosis and incorporate it into his/her daily life. They must acknowledge that they are not like their peers, and that they have a medical condition they will live with for the rest of life. They must begin to think about themselves as people with ADD, and how they will accept this diagnosis. This will give them a sense of their future. You may need to think about changing your job if you feel the need. This decision should not be taken lightly. They need to have a serious assessment done by professional caregivers. The support of family and friends is also important. The individual deciding who to tell and what they say about the diagnosis is their decision. It is sometimes helpful for an adult ADDer, or their supervisor, to explain to their employer or professor and request some of the benefits they may be entitled to.

Another aspect of acceptance is how they view themselves. The ADDer needs to be able to complete any additional training.

This training must include acceptance of their diagnosis and willingness to learn from it. This is often a time when the ADDer must leave behind the comforts and acceptance of their current life to make way for a new, more challenging life.

People

After this assimilation process is complete, the ADDer needs to be honest and admit that they now have a troublesome neurological condition. The consequences of the illness could be made known to their family, friends, coworkers and co-workers. This would help them to accept and be accommodated. They could continue with their normal lives, knowing that they now have ADD. Learning about ADD is a two-way conversation. The ADDer must own their illness and the other must help them in whatever way they can. Sometimes this assistance can be as simple as accepting them as are and giving them lots of encouragement.

People are often the kingpin of an ADDer's growth, development, assimilation into a new reality. Sometimes employers will accept workers with ADD and help them to be more productive by changing their work environment and processes. There are many cases of adults with ADD making subtle improvements to their lives that benefit everyone. These changes are often made after the ADDer leaves their job and is fed up with living under a boss.

I notified my family members, my Western Medical Clinic partners and my colleagues as well the hospital. I was granted admission and had no problems with my staff or at the hospital. The ideas in the book were not something I knew about at the moment of my diagnosis, and they were never implemented by myself. It was not even something I thought of when I was first diagnosed. I must also admit that I am not someone to emulate in terms of the treatment and assimilation process for my ADD.

A New Beginning

All of these changes need to be integrated into a new, better life for the ADDer. This new life might require support from more than the medical team. It may also involve the help of a wider team such as psychologists, sociologists or coaches. It is a good idea to join a local ADD support club, or attend an ADD conference in order to meet other ADDers.

These changes can often take many months, if not years, to become reality. These changes often produce remarkable results. The ADDer develops a new personality and accepts the traits and habits that come with ADD.

I was able to create a support network in Brandon for adults with ADD. This was one of the best things that happened to me. Now, as I am writing this book I realize how much I have struggled to integrate myself into the society. It is a good thing for people with ADD to realize this. Don't regret doing what I did.

Next, we will look at treatment options for ADD.

Chapter 5: Treatments To Add

Every book on ADD that I have ever read has included significant chapters regarding the medical treatment. You should read all of them. You can also search YouTube and Google for ADD or adult ADD. All of these links, especially ones via the Internet need to be interpreted in relation to truth and usefulness.

I find it common for people to jump in too quickly when discussing treatment. However, I would recommend a different approach to helping someone first discover they have ADD. Acceptance, openness to therapy or coaching, followed by medication is what I recommend. We'll explore this in greater detail in the next chapter.

Acceptance

I believe the most important thing in treating ADDer is to make sure they know what it is and that they accept the diagnosis. Acceptance of ADD implies that they don't try to hide their condition or act out. They decide what to accept and which to change. They can choose who and how much they wish to discuss. They should be open and honest about any ADD symptoms they may have. It is important to be open about your diagnosis. While I do not recommend you tell anyone or anything about your diagnosis, it is your decision. However, I advise anyone suffering from ADD to not conceal their symptoms. Instead, they should make every effort to control their behavior as it relates.

Let me explain. The effects of years of being negative and constantly told about your inadequacies, stupidity, and other shortcomings can lead to scarring that can make you feel like you are inferior and damaged goods. The illness has forced you to accept all of your shortcomings, and your inability to understand ADD can lead you towards feeling inferior. Acceptance of your circumstances requires that the ADDer reevaluate their self-image. You must challenge and change their negative view of yourself. You may have a poor work record or have been fired repeatedly for making ignorant statements. Maybe you have a drug problem or alcohol problem that was treated and managed. Accept it all as part of the past. Although you won't mention them to anyone, they will be aware that these problems are part of your history. You accept that these problems were likely to have occurred due to ADD. But, it doesn't necessarily mean you are a bad person. It's just that you are dealing with a condition.

Those who are newly diagnosed with ADD have to come to terms and accept the fact that they are ADD. Sari Solden explains clearly in Journeys Through ADDulthood what it takes to overcome this fear. She shows you how to make someone accept yourself and have fun with your life. Sometimes, it takes years for patients to change their lives.

Personally, I didn't try to make drastic and significant changes in either my personal or professional life after being diagnosed with ADD. I accepted the medical diagnosis and felt that my ADD was fine mentally. I'm ashamed to say that the diagnosis was sometimes used as an excuse for my worst behaviours.

Openness

Your condition should not be hidden. However, you shouldn't try to make it worse. If you make a mistake or are involved in an accident, you must acknowledge that it is there. If you find this difficult to do, you can seek help from a coach. Their job is to ensure you stay on the right track and complete all tasks on time. All young adults suffering from ADD should have support available, particularly if they need it while away at work or school. It is not unusual for university students with ADD abandon their studies just weeks after they arrive at university. For someone with ADD the difference in success or failure can be as simple as asking tough questions.

Your decision about whether to notify your employer and coworkers is up to them, but I recommend being totally honest. This is especially true when dealing with higher education institutions or universities. Many times, these institutions have legislation that will assist you with taking exams and studying.

You should also encourage your support staff members and give them advice. People will not change if we make fun of them or chastise them. Positive encouragement and positive advice can be very helpful.

I was open with my feelings and often blamed my ADD for my tardiness. I didn't learn from my diagnosis and didn't take any steps to correct many of them. I still struggle with procrastination and am shocked at how long this habit has continued.

Therapy and Coaching

Before we begin to look at medications to treat ADD, let's discuss and confirm the benefits of coaching and/or psychotherapy. Highly trained psychotherapists almost exclusively work with people with ADD. To great effect, psychotherapists often employ cognitive behavioural techniques (CBT).

Coaches who are specialized in working with ADDers may be able to instil positive changes in the behavior of adults with ADD. I heard of prominent ADD executives running their own businesses who were being coached to make significant behavioural improvements that improved their lives.

A negative aspect of coaching, private education, and private psychological training is the cost. Many people with adult ADD are not able to afford these specialized professionals. An individual with ADD can improve many of its side effects with the help of educational and medical information.

A community-based ADD/learning disability group is another great place to find support. They meet often and offer great support to those with ADD.

I should have been more interested in my ADD, and its treatment. I don't know why, but I do see it now. Due to other commitments, I didn't have the time or resources to oversee my ADD. My adult ADD symptoms could have been managed if I had received training and planned. These could have included coaching, mentoring and perhaps additional medication. Once the processes are in place it is up to the ADDer if they wish to accept or reject the plan. These processes weren't even considered by me. This is why I wrote this book so that someone else doesn't make the exact same mistake.

Medication

Let's now examine the medication options available to treat adult ADD. These drugs fall into different categories:

* Stimulants

* Non-stimulants

* Antidepressants and other antidepressants

* Hypertensives

* Anticonvulsants

Stimulants

The stimulants that are used for ADD
treatment have been around for a while
and have been thoroughly researched for
their side effects and uses. They have a
bad reputation among the lay population.
They are, in fact, one of the more safe
medications prescribed for psychiatry.
These drugs can no longer be misused.

The first is methylphenidate (represented
by Ritalin, Concerta), which is the second
group of stimulant drug drugs. The other
stimulants include Dexedrine (Adderall),
and Vyvanse (now Vyvanse).

One of the most essential drugs for the
treatment and prevention of ADD is
Ritalin. Dexedrine (Dexedrine), and
Adderall (Adderall), both prescription

stimulant medications can be misused. Both the former are used for high-speed driving and the latter as a sedative.

The goal of stimulant drugs is treatment of ADDers for their attention, alertness memory and concentration. Sometimes stimulant drugs can be used to address ADDer's behavioural problems, such as impulsivity.

The measured results determine the dosage. It is sometimes prescribed in a long acting formulation that lasts for at least 12 hours. If multiple doses are taken, it is recommended that the second dose not be taken before lunch in order to let the ADDer go to sleep at night.

Methylphenidate or Ritalin is the most commonly prescribed stimulant to ADD patients, both for children and adults. Trial and error over a lengthy period is required to determine the right dose.

Side effects of stimulants include anxiety, irritability or muscular tics. These drugs do not cause strokes or heart attacks.

Non-Stimulants

Atomoxetine or Strattera is the main nonstimulant. This drug was initially used as an antidepressant. It was then reintroduced for ADD. Due to the fact that this drug is not a stimulant it has less stringent prescribing requirements.

Antidepressants

Tricyclic antidepressants (MOI, MOI and SSRIs) are the top antidepressants for treating ADD. It is quite amazing to acknowledge that we do not fully understand how antidepressants function. I remember my medical school professors saying, "Use them, and we will figure out their methods of action later!"

Antidepressants of a Different Kind

Atypical antidepressants, a subset of antidepressants that have not been extensively studied, are drugs that work in a way different to regular antidepressants. A number of these atypical drugs have been used to treat ADD. Their side effects are minimal and they have excellent therapeutic results. Wellbutrin HCL (bupropion) is an excellent example. To aid in quitting smoking, the drug is also sold under another name. The medication I've been using for the past ten year is Wellbutrin.

Antihypertensive

The mainstay of antihypertensives used to treat ADD are beta-blockers. Clonidine can also been prescribed. Multimodal presentations of antihypertensives, such as injections, injections, and topical applications, are often an advantage.

Anticonvulsants

Anticonvulsants, the last of the major groups of medicines that may be prescribed for ADD, are also available. These medications are often prescribed together with stimulants. They also help to reduce some of the unacceptable behavioural side effects associated with ADD. You might experience side effects like klazomania or echolalia. All these effects are related to speech sounds and speech. Echolalia can be described as the uncontrolled repetition of words by another person. Coprolalia refers to repetitive swearing. Clazomania is compulsive screaming, and it can come in the form swearing, grunting and barking.

Although I don't intend to make this text a medical reference, I suggest that you check out these three books if there is more information you need about how to prescribe medication to treat ADD.

* Taking Charge of Adult ADHD, Russell A. Barkley. PhD

* Healing ADD, Dr Daniel G. Amen MD

* Driven by Distraction series by Drs. Hallowell and Ratey

Please note that you can access countless videos and articles by these authors on YouTube for no cost.

My medication journey was more accidental than actually prescribed. Discussions about ADD existed in the early days of my diagnosis. There were few authorities, especially in rural Manitoba. I made a mistake and stopped Ritalin before it had time to stabilize in me.

I got well enough to be treated by a psychiatrist who recommended Wellbutrin. It was, unsurprisingly, the best treatment. I have been taking it for close to ten years. This antidepressant is the mainstay in therapy for my type 5 ADD or limbic ADD. A low self-esteem can be associated with depression. Bupropion, which is also sold under the brand Wellbutrin, is recommended as the best treatment.

In the next chapter we will look at the characteristics that are associated with ADD.

Chapter 6: Add Signs, Symptoms And Traits

Many of the professionals who work with people with ADD think that many of the symptoms and signs they experience should be called characteristics. Traits are long-standing, stable behaviours that are not symptomatic of ADD.

The four behavior I am referring to are ADD (Preservation. I'll explain how each trait affects someone with attention problems. I'll talk about its advantages and disadvantages. I'll talk about how the trait manifests itself for the ADDer who is proactive managing their ADD. The trait is also something I personally experienced, both before and after I was diagnosed with ADD.

Preservation

The trait known as preservation allows the ADDer keep on the same path and not stray too far from the goal. To be committed, even in face of great adversity. A preservation trait has the significant benefit of sticking to a goal, and eventually reaching it regardless of what obstacles are in the way. The con to the preservation trait is that you might be unable to do what you want or be able to keep doing it. One example of this is if you refuse to enter a burning building or if you are learning how to play at a sport after a serious injury (although there are some athletes who can play with no limbs).

I doubt I would have ever been able to qualify as a doctor if my ADD had not included the preservation trait. To get into university, it took me about ten more years than I did to leave secondary school. However, I was determined to attend medical school to become a doctor. This attribute of ADD kept my going through medical school, despite any obstacles.

Even though my first wife had a terminal diagnosis, I continued my studies. Even after failing my second MB. I had the need to complete another year of studies, which increased my time at university from six years to seven. This ability to preserve my knowledge allowed me to complete ten years of university studies after I graduated high school. I was determined to attend medical school and become doctor.

This ten year span from the time I left high school to enter university at the young age of 28 (though fellow students were only 18 and 19 respectively) is easily explicable. Dr Russell Barkley's book Taking Charge of Adult ADHD states that the chronological year of a person suffering from ADD is not the actual age. Rightly, he argues that ADDers are only two-thirds their actual chronological age. This explains why traffic accidents are more common in 18-years-olds with ADD.

I realized long before being diagnosed with ADD that if I had entered university when I was 18 years old (rather than 28), I would have absolutely bombed out. I reached adulthood through this extended period of growth, ten years of hard work, and the subsequent university experience. I am grateful to my parents for all their kindness and generosity. Anne, my first spouse, was generous enough to let me attend medical school if it was possible.

Procrastination

Procrastination simply means that someone with ADD has a tendency to delay starting or completing a vital activity.

This is a trait that I believe has no merit. Delaying or even putting off things that are necessary is demoralizing for the individual doing it, and extremely irritating to all others.

Procrastination, which is one of the most irritating, frustrating, and aggravating issues that I have with my ADD, is one of my biggest problems. Procrastination over all kinds of activities and duties is something that causes me to often feel the effects. For example, my wife asked me when I would take the dog out for a stroll and the kids wanted to know when McDonald's was open. I'd reply to both, but then I'd forget about the plan and get on with something else.

Procrastination can be more severe when there are multiple bills that must be paid electronically. I can get so focused on other things that I forget to pay bills. It's fascinating to note that I never had procrastination at work, even in the ER.

Sandra, my wife, deserves to be commended for her patience and willingness to let me put off doing things around the house that I promised. There are many ways to do this. Some examples include taking the dog out for a walk, getting the mail and putting away the garbage.

Another extension of my procrastination is that I suddenly change my mind. I have a five-minute time limit for taking the dog for a walk, but by the end of the five minutes I am putting the garbage out. Or when I'm driving, I decide to take the children Dairy Queen. However, after changing my mind, I end up at McDonald's. This is my suspicion that my ADD type and my procrastination are responsible for my indecision and mind-changing.

Hyperfocus

Hyperfocus can be a valuable ADD trait if used in the right context. Hyperfocus is when something takes control and all other activities are forgotten. Hyper-focused ADDers may miss meals or even forget to go back to sleep until they crash.

This hyperfocus ability is very helpful in many situations at work. If a person with ADD can identify the activities that cause them to be hyperfocused, they may be able to find a job or a new career. An example of this would be a judge, comedian or police officer. These are just a few examples.

A person with hyperfocus has a lot of advantages. It can have a tremendous impact on both the ADDer, and the subject or task that is causing hyperfocus. Hyperfocus is when an ADDer hyper focuses their attention on dangerous behaviour. The immediate examples of this would be abuse of drugs, alcohol, and sex.

Hyperfocus has been a tool I use in many medical situations. It's also helpful when driving as it gives me the ability to drive fast while being aware of everything around me. This aspect of my awareness is not as sharp as it used to be when I was younger.

Impulsivity

Injuries and serious accidents often occur in childhood, particularly teens. ADD causes serious accidents because the child does not have any idea of danger or fear. As we age, our abilities to count to 10 become more sophisticated. Adult impulsivity is both a blessing as well as a curse.

The pro of impulsivity means the ability to take immediate action and make decisions without conscious thought to control a situation.

Inimpulsivity is a common problem. It's when an immediate action is taken that leads to a mistake. This is often the case in situations of extreme drama. We are seeing numerous complaints about police abuses, and the shootings of innocent people of color. You can see that these situations are stressful and it is not an acceptable reactionary behavior. If the person who committed the act has ADD, it would be part of the impulsivity.

I have been guilty of many impulsive actions that led to me in serious trouble. However, the consequences were not severe. Here is an example I have of impulsivity in my life. My family and myself moved into a house and were unpacking all of our stuff and trying make order. My wife was furious about my procrastination regarding clearing out the utility rooms. When I went down to clean it, I noticed a large cardboard bag containing many old and cheap frames. It was from my office at the clinic. They had been laying around for a long time, but they were empty. I clearly remember throwing the container out. Months later, the box contained my Dundee University certificate that stated that I had passed my exam to become a medical doctor. After much research, I was fortunate enough to find a notarized copy of my certificate which I have used as needed.

This is related to my impulsivity. When I am waiting in a long queue, I find that it is difficult for me to keep my cool. I have noticed that I often get frustrated easily and take stupid actions or do stupid stuff. I'll swear for several seconds after the computer does something wrong. Then, it will go back to normal. I do this often when watching TV. Then another stupid commercial that has been shown a thousand times is on again. This causes instant irritation and allows me to return to normal. Perhaps the worst aspect is my impulsive anger when driving. Even though another driver annoys and disturbs me, it's not a problem. I swear and then I'm back to normal in a matter of seconds.

ADD can lead to four distinct symptoms or traits: preservation, hyperfocus and procrastination. These are the four most annoying traits that I have observed in myself. As you can see, preservation and hyperfocus both have pros and cons. However, I am unable to find any pros about procrastination.

The next chapter will examine three of my "con," or what I call my deficient states (DS).

Chapter 7: Time: My First Defective State

In my own experiences with ADD, certain affective state have been observed in me, something I mentioned in chapter 4. To briefly review: what I call "affective states" can either be positive--"effective" or negative--"defective". An ADDer's ability to perceive a particular issue as an affective state. As I saw it myself, positive (or even effective) states for ADDers are those that focus on education, family, and personal interests. In another book, I will explore these positive states more. I am dedicating a chapter to each of three negative (defective), states I have encountered. These are my thoughts about money, time management, and possessions. Although I can't connect ADD with my dysfunctional relationship with these states, I believe it plays a part.

I'll try to explain why and how I got there. First, time management is my DS. The next two I will be discussing are money (financial), or possessions. I intend to discuss the impact ADD has on these states. I have described these deficient states in an effort to raise awareness of ADD among those with ADD and their family members, friends, and supporters.

Time management was the first defect I experienced, something I suspect many with ADD have to struggle with. Is it time management that is so difficult to manage for ADDers? There are many theories. You can think of it this way: Time exists only in two ways for someone with ADD. They have to choose between "now" or not now. Recent research has shown that ADDers perceive the world as a series of events rather than sequentially as do people without ADD. Another research suggests that ADDers have "time blindness", which means they live in a perpetual state where they are always late. These descriptions indicate that ADDers may have a distorted perspective of time.

Because of their distorted idea of time, it may make sense that the ADDer is always late. It is possible that the ADDer makes incorrect predictions about the duration of various tasks. This can also lead to a distorted view of time. The ADDer needs to be able realistically plan for long term projects. However, it is likely that the ADDer will struggle to stick to the plan.

I remember the fourth year project that I did in medical school. I spent many hours researching this project over the course of several weeks. However, I failed to realize how much time it took me to create the report. Although my teacher gave me a pass grade, he also knew how extensive I was researching. However, I believe I should have received an A if the report had been written in the appropriate time.

The ADDer's distorted perception of time is a result of the traits described in the chapter on Preservation, Procrastination Hyperfocus and Impulsivity. What I've found is that when I'm completing a task but it's time for another, I feel the overwhelming need to do one more thing before moving onto the next item on my schedule. This urge to do yet another task continues. It becomes so much that I dedicate way, way too much of my time to the task at hand, and my day's plan is completely disrupted. Could this be hyperfocus? What about impulsivity-- impulsively daring to do just one more thing (over and over again)? Perhaps there is a link between the trait of procrastination (failing to complete tasks on time) and impulsivity. Maybe preservation plays into this a too strong devotion, almost even a compulsion? To continue pursuing the given job despite the fact that it is not in the schedule, and it would make more sense to the rest of the ADDer's day, week or month. I think these are classic traits that contribute to ADDer's time management problems.

My inability to stay on schedule and my struggle with TM began when it was my responsibility as a teenager for me to get up at the right time to get to school. As a teenager, I was responsible for my own time and struggled to manage it. This led to my struggles with TM that continued for decades. I was always late at school, struggled with the TMC in my work life after high school, but I never considered it a problem. Strange though this may seem, it was for me.

I had to seriously question my time management skills when I spoke with engineers in an Edinburgh hotel bar. I had a great conversation with them, and they explained how they could hand work over to someone else while still being on time. I was in the midst of my thirties. I was a sixth grade medical student. I was also doing locum home officer jobs. I was experiencing difficulty leaving my job on the scheduled date. I still remember the conversation as a result of which engineers could not comprehend my problem. Transferring duties was a constant problem for me. It was a problem that recurred again when I went to general practice and entered the jam-packed emergency rooms. Because I tried to tidy up any loose ends, I was usually an hour to one hour and half late to go home. It was also a problem that I was always a little late to start my shift. I called the ER every day, right after my scheduled time, to say, "I'm up the North Hill, will get there in five minute!"

As you can see, I struggle to accurately assess how long it will be me to complete a task. My example is calling my wife and saying, "I will be on my way back in a few moments." Only one more patient is needed. After a quick interview with the patient and a simple exam, prescription renewal and examination, they may mention something in passing as they leave. The conversation can go on for up to an hour. This was a routine occurrence for me as a GP. Sometimes I was just a few minutes late with a few patients.

Let me offer an example. Say I had Raymond, a patient. Raymond would be walking out of the room and mention that his hunting rifle had been purchased. I might then ask him if Raymond is a hunter. Raymond might tell me that he is not a hunter after I encourage him. In this situation, all time is lost. I have to then deal with the situation and involve his family and friends. This comment may not add an extra hour to a patient appointment, but it is something that would occur often. Many patients also requested repeat prescriptions and wanted to talk about additional issues. You may also be asked to call your doctor or visit you at home. Before leaving my office, however, I had the responsibility of reviewing all laboratory results and arranging urgent referrals. I rarely left my office at 5 p.m., but more like 7:30 p.m.

As a GP, I ran more and more behind in the mornings and afternoons. I also used to go out for coffee every afternoon while patients waited for me. I believe this was my way of dealing with my ADD. Also, it broke up a very long session within the office. This allowed for me to continue working in a busy, stressful group practice. I sincerely apologize to all the patients and staff that were adversely affected by my lack of consideration and poor manners.

My children also suffered from my TM problem. When we first arrived to Canada from Scotland, my son encouraged me to play soccer with him. I attempted coaching. I gave up because of my poor timekeeping. Also, I have to admit that my resignation was probably for the team's good!

Because of my poor time management, I quit as a GP/FP to become an EMO at the Brandon General Hospital.

Surprisingly I found some improvements in my time management after I became a civilian medic officer at the local military camp at age 70. We started at 7:30 am and the sick parade was at 8:30 am. Working with the military meant that I had to follow orders. I started changing the way I managed my time. I got up at 5:30

AM, left the house by 7:00 AM, and was at work at the time set. It was clear to me that if my alarm went off before 7:00, I would arrive at work on-time. Because of the many years I spent serving in the military, it was through these years that I learned the value of scheduling my time and following that plan. I finally learned how to make changes and stay on time.

I am now surprisingly punctual and on time for most of the appointments. I take my wife regularly to the Brandon cancer care facility. With her encouragement, we never leave home late.

With my amazing success in turning around almost six decades worth of struggles with time management, at the age of seventy-eight, I see this as a way to bring hope to fellow ADDers. This is what I would tell other ADDers. I wish this advice had been given to me earlier. Like the many difficulties that ADDers face, we need to be vigilant about how our time is managed. We need to remember that we are poor at managing our time. This is why it is so important to prepare for all possible consequences when we judge time. Additional aids like a smartphone or a timer, calendar or personal diary can be very helpful. It is up to us how we arrange our lives in a way that makes it possible to review our commitments, make proper plans, and stick to the program.

I believe it is vital for us ADDers to plan our days and set up what is necessary. It is important to set a time and stick to it. Accept that you'll be late sometimes, forgive yourself, then get back on track with your plan. Don't be discouraged by your inability to keep time. Be proactive, but don't beat yourself up about timekeeping.

Now let's get to the money.

Chapter 8: Money - The Second Of My Defective States

Financial planning (FP)--money--is my second defective state. My Achilles heel in the area of managing money is financial planning. My Achilles heel is the ADDer's impulsivity and disregard for the future makes it difficult for us to find appropriate strategies to ensure proper financial management.

ADDers are known for making plans but never following through. Our ADD symptoms constantly interfere with our efforts for change. For me, this meant that I didn't do my FP correctly or on the right time. I wasn't consistent or regular in saving and spending. Adult ADDers find it more difficult to manage their spending. These traits are detrimental to ADDers' efforts to save for the long-term and prevent a "rainy night" situation.

Unfortunately, money management involves a lot of steps and processes, which is why ADDers are so afraid to do it. The whole process for managing money is against the will of ADDers who are constantly struggling. It requires that you have a clear vision about the future. This is impossible, considering what I just wrote in Chapter 1 about our misunderstood notion of time. It also requires that we keep track of income and expenses on a regular basis. Being consistent and consistent with tracking money can be difficult when you have traits like procrastination or impulsivity. But the traits that preserve and hyperfocus show that it is not impossible. I do want to acknowledge one thing. I can confirm that money is a major problem in my own case. Other ADDers may view money in a different way. However, they might feel that money is one of their affective or positive states due to the financial benefits and their experience. As you can see, these affective states are either beneficial or detrimental for the ADDer.

What are the basics of managing money and financial plan? Track all our spending and keep track of our bank accounts balances. Paying the household bills and especially taxes on time--no procrastinating!--otherwise, trouble ensues. Keeping credit cards current and paying them off monthly--again, no procrastinating!--and not using them for impulse purchases. Even though we may not see the future as it is, or at least not in the way we think it will happen, it is important to plan for the present. These are all important processes that need to be performed consistently and accurately, with all the required additional requirements. However, they can be difficult for ADDers.

My financial problems started 18 months after my family arrived in Canada. At that time, I was presented with a cheque for $2,000. It was from my cousin and lawyer in Glasgow. This was the money I got from selling my home here in Scotland. I had planned to make $20,000 from the house's sale, but was wrongly assuming that. You will see that I severely underestimated.

My financial problems worsened after I started my practice. Due to unpaid taxes, Revenue Canada placed us in debt. In order to pay the taxes, I borrowed funds. In order to pay the taxes, every year it seemed I'd need to borrow money from a bank. Thanks to my wife's tremendous support and encouragement, we are now free from debt with Revenue Canada. Without her continued support and assistance, I wouldn't have achieved this. I have been overpaying taxes for years and only getting the occasional check back.

A long time ago, I was driving with a Rotary member who was an investor salesman. He pointed out that, given my income, I should be putting aside $1,000 per month. I clearly remember telling him that I couldn't manage $100. I would often look at the numbers, try to understand them, then attempt to resolve the debt. It is obvious that I have arranged a revolving loan of credit. Although the credit limit has been reduced over time, it is still not completely clear. Due to my higher earning capacity, it has been a difficult decision to allow myself to remain in debt for a while. I had no idea the long-term consequences of this. This is because I overspent regularly. I overspent but should have saved. I did not take the proper action.

Many times, I was advised to change my bad habits over the years. Another example of advice is when I reached out to a financial adviser in the United States. She kindly called me Saturday morning, many years ago, and advised that I get out my debt. A Royal Bank agent suggested the same thing, but I refused to listen because he spoke in a belligerent manner. I instead closed my account and moved to another bank. I'm sorry to say that my ADD was directing how I reacted at the time. I could have understood and followed his recommendations had the agent been more helpful.

I'm well aware of the fact that impulse shopping has been a significant problem for my health and that it's difficult to manage. I only realized how much I had spent on all manner of things after I retired. I bought tools that were never used, magazines and books that were never reread, and I bought cards and presents that I never appreciated. Only purchase and spend after careful consideration of the cost-benefit ratio. Not at your whim or impulsivity.

CME, also known as continuing medical education (CME), is one expense that doctors must pay. CME/CPD is combined with all my professional licenses (and insurance) cost me more than $1,500 per month to continue in practice. These conferences were a way for my wife to see more of her new country.

In recent years, we have been enjoying cruising as a relaxing and enjoyable form of vacation. Cruising is a luxury that we both enjoy. It was one of the things that allowed us to relax and unwind after a stressful life. Cruising has allowed us the opportunity to visit many places in Europe, Russia (the Middle East), Asia, Alaska, Hawaii, West Indies, Panama Canal, North and South America. Many of these travels have been made since my wife's diagnosis with lung cancer. These cruises also bring up another aspect in all the financial woes. The good times, the excitement and reward of raising a family and integrating all of us into the Canadian way to live are just some of the many. Looking back at all we have accomplished, it makes me realize that we have not done too badly.

Why didn't my budget work? I tried unsuccessfully many budgets and other expenses plans. None of these seemed to work for me as I was suffering undiagnosed adult ADD. I tried multiple techniques for different periods and none worked. It required constant input throughout the day. I discovered a new approach to budgeting, the "One-Number Strategy", more recently. This strategy requires you to identify four monthly expenses. Add all four expenses together and subtract your monthly take-home income. Divide this number by the number days in a given month. This is your "one numbers". It's the money you have available to spend every day. This money can go towards entertainment, shopping, clothes, hobbies and other purposes. However, you are not allowed borrow in advance. You can however accumulate cash to pay for large expenses. The only problem with this budget is that it was discovered during COVID-19. Not when I was making regular monthly salaries, but when I was becoming redundant. I didn't realize I needed this budget when I was working.

I hadn't realized I was getting old until the last 18months. Maybe it was my bad time management. This was also a factor in my failure to save money for the long-term. I suspect this was due to the ADD-related inhibition of executive function.

I was doing research on financial planning and came across this quote from Jim Rohn. This is how I feel.

"There will be two types of pain in your life.

The pain of discipline and regret

Discipline is worth a few ounces; regret, on the other hand, can be worth a lot.

I'd be pleased if my complete inability to develop a financial plan can help one person with ADD or not to change their destructive money management behavior. Let me finish by offering some hard-earned wisdom: Track your spending and get a good idea of your bank balances. It is important to pay all bills, including taxes, on time. Don't make impulse purchases, keep your credit cards current and pay them off each month. You should save for the future.

The next chapter will be about possession. Irresponsible spending to obtain these items is the cause. It all comes down to ADD although I am not entirely sure how.

Chapter 9: Possessions 3: The Third Of My Deficitive States

Possessions is the third of my many deficient states, and the last one we'll discuss. I've seen the accumulation of possessions in my life. This is a state I know to be defective. I wonder if the ADDer is suffering from impaired executive functioning (EF). This loss in EF can lead to disinhibition. It causes a failure to pay attention to the problem.

The trait of impulsivity, which is the tendency to buy more stuff, can be attributed to the accumulation of too much stuff. It could also refer to hyperfocus or preservation, where I can be so focused and focused on a task that any item, material, or thing related to it, without having to think about whether I have the item in question or not.

When I refer to "possessions", or "stuff", that means a ratbag of different objects and things that have been accumulated indirectly or directly. The accumulation of stuff is strongly linked to my ADD. For a moment, imagine the untidy desk of an ADDer. It is full of papers and files. My desk is not the only one.

My office stuff consists of files on my desk, piles in the bookcase, and paper. These files include plans, ideas, and projects I've tried and abandoned. Some of these ventures included an Amazon seller account and a Shopify Store. I was enthusiastic about both but gave up on them. This whole process of finding a project and becoming passionate about it, as well as doing extensive research and spending lots of money and time, is something I've repeated time and again. This behavior is common among ADDers. For me, the project is often educational in nature, and sometimes medical. However,

I see it as a financial scheme that can help me get rich quickly.

Our house is home to many different magazines. Many of them are medical and include National Geographic, Discovery, Rotarian, Maclean's, Maclean's, National Geographic, Discovery, Rotarian, and Discovery. They get thrown out, or given to a personal assistance home every so often. This cleaning is something that I don't do very often. Sandra must insist on it.

My clothing as well as my footwear is another source of stuff. I have been able to reduce the number of shoes that I own and keep it under control. The same can be said about the number of suits or trousers I own, and the amount of shirts I have. Although I have to admit that I used to not associate my mass clothes with ADD until recently I now realize that the two are part and parcel of what I view as a hoarding disorder.

The utility room has shelves and an under-stair cupboard that can hold more stuff. These areas can house an old computer as well as electronic parts and a box of paper.

The garage has shelves that hold many more boxes that have items from Scotland. Other shelves include tools, painting supplies, and wall-hanging paraphernalia. Overall, the garage is untidy and full of stuff. One positive is the fact that the loft area I built above it to store even more stuff is now empty. At least it is for now.

Since childhood, I've had a problem with stuff. It was something that I noticed only after I was diagnosed as having ADD. My mother had the exact same problem. Both of us accumulate stuff in piles and containers in our office areas, garages and garden sheds.

Me and My Gunnysack

Although I carry a "gunnysack", which is more commonly a briefcase these days, it was actually a bag I carried with me to work in the past. It contained a lot of things that I believed I would need, such as a prescription pad, stethoscope, sphygmomanometer (blood pressure measuring machine), tendon hammer, etc. This bag contained some general medical references and a few tools that I would use, including a prescription pad, stethoscope (blood pressure measuring machine), tendon Hammer, etc. All these pieces of equipment were always on hand in my consultation room. But, even though I knew I would need them, I felt the need to have back-up materials. So, I always had a spare Stethoscope. A prescription pad, surgical gloves and a notepad. The need to keep these items around my work area, including the garage, home, and most importantly my home office, would appear completely redundant. If I did not have my gunnysack filled with redundant items, it would make me feel inept and unequipped to carry out my duties. This is almost like these items are a badge of honor that affirms my identity as a doctor. I suspect this feeling, and this need, are related to my ADD. The gunnysack serves as a badge and a crutch for me to maintain my professionalism.

Over the years, many times I tried to limit or remove my gunnysack. This would cause me anxiety. I resolved this by reconnected with my gunnysack. My gunnysack enabled me to confirm my profession before I could perform my duties comfortably.

Another interesting aspect of accumulation and duplication over the years is the amount it has cost. It reached an extreme level when I discovered that I had nine different pairs of headphones. They were spread throughout the house and could not be gathered together.

Possibly to some readers, it doesn't seem that the collection of things has any relation with the diagnosis of ADD. I don't think there are any links between accumulation and ADD. There is no correlation between them in my particular situation. According to the Mayo Clinic's prestigious clinic, hoarding is due to indecisiveness or perfectionism. These symptoms all directly correlate to the diagnosis of ADD. This realization about my hoarding tendencies as well as my accumulation of stuff gives me some relief.

Let me finish by saying that even though I collect stuff, I am not an over-accumulator. Don't get the impression that my house is full with junk. It's very clean and comfortable, but it's full of junk.

Chapter 10: Adult Adhd: Myths And Symptoms

Understanding ADHD and its effects on your daily life is essential for managing adult ADHD. ADHD sufferers often fall into the trap of thinking negative about their ability to manage everyday tasks and perform simple tasks. These behaviors are often caused by ADHD symptoms. It is possible to let go of the negative emotions and instead work with ADHD.

It can be difficult to recognize symptoms even for people who suspect they may have adult ADHD. Adult ADHD can be misunderstood and misinterpreted. In addition, misinformation can lead to a rise in stigma about mental health disorders. This will further alienate those who are already struggling to live up to society's expectations. These myths are a major deterrent to people seeking help, getting diagnosed and receiving the treatment they require.

The confusion around adult ADHD can make some mistake their behavior for adult ADHD symptoms. Many people have trouble focusing on tasks that are tedious or not interesting. Many others struggle with time management and organization. The behavior of adults with ADHD is markedly different. It's both disruptive and genetically induced. Let's clear up some confusion about adult ADHD.

What is adult ADHD and what are its symptoms?

Attention Deficit/hyperactive Disorder (ADHD), is a neurochemical imbalance that affects the ability of sufferers to focus on tasks, prioritize and organize their lives, and have a calm, focused disposition. ADHD often begins in childhood. The symptoms usually disappear with age.

ADHD symptoms can persist into adulthood and adolescence for many people. About 70% of ADHD sufferers continue to experience symptoms through adolescence. Half of them also experience them into adulthood.

Many people with ADHD don't get diagnosed until they become adults. This could be because they didn't know it was there all their lives. Although doctors do not know exactly what causes ADHD, experts believe genetic disposition, early exposure to lead, and infancy exposure to toxic substances such as drugs and cigarettes may all play a part.

ADHD is caused in part by an abnormal brain function that blocks neurotransmitter dopamine from reaching the brain. When this happens, the reward system in the brain is blocked, which means that those with ADHD don't get the same neurochemical benefits as those without it. ADHD sufferers will seek out experiences that increase their dopamine levels to make up the deficit. ADHD sufferers need constant stimulation and new experiences to release dopamine. This makes it hard to focus on tasks without immediate reward.

Psychostimulants and other drugs are prescribed often by psychiatrists. They help to redirect brain chemicals to where they need them to. Prescription treatment is often successful for many people, but it's not always the best. Before you start or stop taking prescriptions, talk with your doctor.

The symptoms

While every adult ADHD sufferer experiences symptoms differently, the majority of ADHD symptoms are similar. The signs are more severe in males than they are for females. As children, males are more likely to be hyperactive. They may not be able slow down and concentrate. As we age, the symptoms generally disappear.

Women may not experience symptoms until puberty, when hormones change brain chemistry. ADHD can manifest in different ways for men. For example, ADHD may be experienced more frequently as disorganization and forgetfulness in women.

All symptoms are experienced by people of both genders. Here are the symptoms of ADHD as an adult:

* Extreme difficulty staying organized, due to inability or unwillingness to focus on tasks. This causes missed appointments, unpaid bill, missed deadlines, and loss of important items like keys, wallets or cell phones.

* Issues related to prioritizing tasks

* Poor planning skills.

* Having difficulty starting tasks.

* You are easily distracted and find it difficult to focus on the important tasks.

* Impulsiveness. This can lead to dangerous situations when ADHD people engage in reckless behavior.

* Often being late.

* Poor listening skills.

* Trouble listening and honoring commitments can lead to problems in relationships.

* Sudden mood swings/outbursts.

* Being easily frustrated and hot-tempered.

* Trouble coping stress.

* Restlessness and difficulty sleeping or relaxing.

* Learning disabilities.

* Low self esteem.

* ADHD may be accompanied with anxiety or depression.

Myths

It is not clear how myths began, but mental illness myths are harmful for both those with the illness and those who care about them. Debunking myths can help you understand your symptoms better and make it easier for others to help you.

The following myths are often associated with adult ADHD. They have been corrected.

ADHD is not considered a medical disorder.

Yes. ADHD can lead to neurobiological symptoms. It is caused by a chemical imbalance.

ADHD isn't a problem.

ADHD is a disability which makes it difficult to perform at the level of people who don't have it. ADHD individuals often require special accommodations to improve their ability to learn and function more efficiently. These accommodations help people with ADHD to succeed. ADHD is a real condition, with symptoms that arise naturally from the neurochemical imbalance in your brain.

ADHD is something that ADHD children will always overcome.

False. It is false. ADHD is often not diagnosed in adults, even if it was recognized as a child's condition. Some also have other mood disorders such anxiety or depression.

ADHD affects boys only.

ADHD can affect males and women equally, although the symptoms are often different between men and females.

ADHD medications turn patients into zombies.

Prescriptions for ADHD are effective in correcting the brain's chemical imbalance when prescribed at the correct dosage. These prescriptions can help increase neurotransmitter receptivity as well as block the transport of dopamine back to the brain's neural cells, thereby increasing brain dopamine. This will help the patient stay calm and focus.

Sometimes, it may take time for both the patient and the doctor to find the dose that is right. Although symptoms can be unpleasant, the adjustment period for any medication that alters the brain's Neurochemistry may cause some discomfort. These should usually only last a few days.

Patients who were hyperactive, restless, impulsive, or hyperactive in the past, will no longer need stimulation. When the chemical imbalance is corrected, they can return to their old behavior. While this may cause a noticeable difference in patient's personality, it is actually a sign that the patient is being treated for medical conditions.

ADHD is the result bad parenting or a lack of discipline during childhood.

ADHD is considered a medical condition. Certain parenting techniques can certainly worsen ADHD symptoms. However, for some patients, hard expectations and discipline cannot help them overcome their symptoms unless accommodations have been made.

Sometimes ADHD symptoms can be disguised with strong structure and organization from parents. Individuals suddenly find it challenging to recreate the organization they have created from their family's early years. This is why ADHD is often not diagnosed until adults. The symptoms of ADHD can not be corrected by the best parenting if the parents do not educate their children on the condition and teach them how to cope.

ADHD patients are either lazy, stupid, or just plain disobedient.

ADHD is a common disorder that affects many people. Many ADHD individuals are intelligent beyond their peers and can excel in their chosen field if they understand how best to meet their needs. They are simply unable to keep their eyes on the longer-term reward and lack of motivation. ADHD people can struggle to reach long-term goals and plan for the future if they don't have immediate payoff.

ADHD patients can be laser-focused for hours on activities that provide a lot of enjoyment and/or constant stimulation. For people to remain focused and motivated, they must learn to work with their reward system.

There are many myths surrounding ADHD. And the details of each person's symptoms are unique. Talking with a psychiatrist or doctor about ADHD can be helpful in clearing up any confusions and digging deeper to identify the many symptoms.

Chapter 11: Simple Strategies For Boosting Productivity

With a good understanding of ADHD symptoms in adulthood, we can now explore ways to cope with the effects of ADHD that extend beyond medication. ADHD symptoms can be treated with accommodations that minimize the impact on your life.

ADHD adults may not be the only ones experiencing problems with productivity. There are many resources available that can help you find time management strategies and productivity hacks. These strategies and tools can work for some people, but they may not be right for everyone. You need to be honest about your situation. These strategies will be more effective if you are aware of your condition, and choose to work with it instead of against it.

Stop Procrastinating

People with ADHD and people without ADHD are both at greatest risk of losing productivity due to procrastination. ADHD people have unique challenges to overcome procrastination. Because their brain is hardwired to be easily distracted, they face unique challenges. ADHD individuals are likely to find excuses to procrastinate easier than others. They must make efforts to stop this behavior.

There are many ways to overcome procrastination when it comes to completing tasks. Do small tasks right away. You should complete tasks that take less than two minutes such as packing up or returning calls immediately. The easier the task, it's more likely that it will get forgotten. A number of uncompleted, small tasks can quickly pile up.

It doesn't matter if you hate a task because it's hard or boring. You should make it a priority to finish it by the time you get up in the morning. It's a good idea to plan ahead for the next day and to make a list with all the steps required to complete the task. If you have a plan, you can start quickly and feel much better after the worst happens.

When you have difficulty starting tasks, make a commitment to spend at least 15 minutes working on them. The task will become less daunting and easier to manage if it is broken down into smaller time periods. To keep track of the time, you can set up a timer. Once the timer goes off you can either stop and take a short break or go on for another 20-minutes. It doesn't matter how small your progress, it will inspire you to keep going.

Prioritize

ADHD people often struggle with prioritizing tasks. But this skill is critical to productivity. Prioritizing ensures that you finish the most critical and urgent tasks first to avoid missing deadlines or failing to complete projects. This questionnaire can help you identify which tasks should be prioritized and which ones should be left to the last.

* Which task is closest to the deadline?

* Which task will take me the longest and require more work?

* Which task, once completed, will make the rest of the tasks easier?

* What are the first tasks I must complete before I can take on more tasks?

* Which tasks can impact the work and performance of others?

* Which tasks take a long time before I can get to them?

Plan Ahead

Once you know your priorities, plan ahead to ensure everything gets done on-time. Whether you use an electronic or paper planner, it will be easier to track all your tasks. You'll also have a visual aid that allows you to prioritize, add tasks, mark completion, and record when things are done.

Each night, prepare for the next day by planning your night before bed. Your tasks and appointments should be listed in the order they will get completed. The week will be planned out on Sunday nights. Make a list of the most important tasks that must be completed and set deadlines. The same process can be done at the start of the month to give you a general overview of your life. You can make sure that everything gets done in a timely manner by doing this.

Establish Routines

Routines are beneficial when you have certain tasks that repeat often. You can make these tasks automatic by creating routines. These tasks are not something you have to think about. Efficiency is all about energy management. The less time you spend making decisions, you will have more energy to focus on and complete tasks.

You must establish habits in order to make your routines stick. Psychologists state that it takes 21 working days to make a habit. This is something you should keep in mind as you begin your routines. You should focus on one or two habits at the time and not try to change everything. It's easier to stick to small steps than to create a routine. You'll also be motivated to do more as you succeed.

Batch Tasks

Even small tasks you must do every day can consume large chunks of your daily time if they are done randomly. Stopping in the middle of a task can cause you to lose precious minutes of your day.

Batching refers the practice or allocating specific time to accomplish tasks of similar difficulty. For example, you might set aside 15 minutes each day to answer email, check social networks, or return phone calls. These tasks will get completed if you set aside a specific time.

Break long tasks into manageable steps

It is easier to break down long tasks into smaller pieces if you have trouble keeping your attention on them. The big picture can become overwhelming. However, it's much more manageable to tackle one task at at time. Plan a project by setting small milestones. Then, reward yourself with an artificial reward each time you complete one of those milestones. For example, you might reward yourself with five minute of social media time, a quick walk, or your favorite healthy food when you have completed a task. This will help you to meet your brain's stimulation needs and compensate for any deficiencies in your neurochemistry's reward systems.

A Distraction-Free Workspace that is Organized and Well-Designed

To keep productivity high, it is crucial to have an organized workspace. It is important to have a clean, organized workspace to maximize productivity. The less time you take to find what you need, the more time you will have to spend on those tasks. It will save you time and help you focus on your other tasks by keeping your email inbox clean, filing important papers away, and organizing your workspace.

It is important to have a space that allows you to focus and maintain a high level. Your phone should not distract you while you are working. To temporarily avoid internet surfing, you can download an app. This will keep you away from sites that are likely to lure you in like social media sites. Your coworkers should not interrupt you while you are working on tasks, except in an emergency. Be respectful of your time and accept that you may not be able to turn down requests when necessary.

Play to your strengths

ADHD doesn't mean that everything is difficult. ADHD may give people an advantage over others in certain situations because of their unique qualities. ADHD individuals can have more energy than others and are therefore better suited for careers or tasks that require them to be productive quickly.

A job that requires you to be hyperfocused on particular details is a good fit for you. You should know your strengths and utilize them when you volunteer or choose the career and job path that suits you best.

Change it if it's not working

Sometimes, it doesn't matter what you do, you just can not make it work. This could be a job you are having trouble with motivation, a college program that isn't holding your attention the way you hoped, or any other situation. This might not be the right job for you. Instead of dwelling on negative thoughts about yourself and how you perform in these endeavors. It's fine if this is true. Even those with ADHD are often not a good fit for their chosen career or area of study.

Allow yourself to make changes if you feel that something isn't working. Change can be difficult, but you should enjoy the excitement of a new environment. You will be surprised at how much you can accomplish if you choose a path that captivates your interest and is within your reach.

Your productivity can be improved by trying different strategies and tools to see which one works for you. Be positive and keep working until you find your productivity sweet place. You will feel so happy once you reach that sweet spot.

Chapter 12: Your Adhd And Your Partner

Adult ADHD is a difficult diagnosis for many people. However, it can be difficult for others to cope with the condition. It can be hard to see the world from another perspective when your own symptoms are so overwhelming. However, this perspective is essential for our well-being, and it's an important step toward self-development.

Relationships that are in conflict can create a lot of tension for both partners. ADHD sufferers will find that stress can lead to more symptoms. This can affect their ability to focus and function in other areas. This can make it worse for relationships, trapping you in a vicious cycle of frustration and miscommunication.

ADHD is best managed through supportive and healthy relationships. For healthy and open relationships to develop, you need to look at things from another perspective. If you are able to understand the symptoms of your partner, it is possible to begin to empathize with them and to open the doors to communication in order to resolve the issues together.

Your partner might feel lonely.

People may feel they aren't listening to you if you have trouble staying focused when others are speaking. If you move around a lot, look around, or interrupt others while they are talking, your partner might feel that you don't care about their words. Intimacy is built on listening and respect. Both partners must be able and willing to listen to their partner.

Sometimes your partner might feel that they are the ones doing all the work.

Even though dirty dishes in the sink and laundry scattered across the bedroom floor are not likely to bother you, it could be a problem for your partner. It may not seem that much, but if your partner is continually picking up the slack they might feel exploited. For a relationship to be balanced and harmonious, both partners should pull their weight equally.

"Doing all work" can also be used to describe the emotional world. They may feel they have to bring up everything when it's time for a conversation. Your partner's emotional needs are just as important as your own.

Sometimes your partner might feel you don't honor your promises.

While you may promise to keep your promises, even if you do so with the best of intentions, your partner will feel like you're not keeping them. To build trust and trust in a relationship it is important to keep your promises and commit to them. If you don't do this, your relationship will quickly crumble.

Your spending habits may cause anxiety in your partner.

When you're in a long-term marriage, the combined finances means that both spouses work together to pay your bills and help to support the household. Both are responsible for budgeting and savings to achieve your goals and keep things running smoothly. But if you spend too much and don't have the discipline to pay your bills on-time, your partner could be continually stressed about finances.

According to research, money is the main reason most couples fight. If you are experiencing constant tension and fights in your relationship, this can lead to a serious strain on the relationship. To keep the household safe and stable, both spouses must adopt responsible money habits.

Sometimes your partner might feel the need to nag and nag you to get any work done.

You may feel stressed if your partner constantly reminds you and asks questions to compensate for your forgetfulness or tardiness. Each partner must be capable of handling their own responsibilities in order to have a mature relationship. It could feel like your partner is taking care of an adult child. You may also feel constantly nag and pestered.

It is important that everyone reminds each other to do the most important domestic tasks. However, if one person is reminding the other all the time and the other is doing all it, tension will undoubtedly reign.

If anger and frustration outbursts are a common occurrence, it could make your partner feel victimized.

People who are easily angered and frustrated will know how difficult it can be to have these outbursts happen regularly. But if you partner is always at the receiving end of your outbursts, they probably won't feel very comfortable with being yelled at. It is important to show patience when two people try to connect their lives.

It is difficult to live with ADHD, but it is possible for a partner to cope with it. Give your partner the same compassion, understanding, and kindness that you would like.

It is possible for your partner to feel unhappy, lonely, and/or depressed.

While you may experience these feelings on your path to managing adult ADHD, it is possible that your partner might also feel this way. It is possible for your partner to feel isolated and lonely if they are too busy dwelling in their own thoughts and not communicating with you. Feeling like they are not being "checked into" and managing your business as an adult can cause them to feel frustrated and isolated.

ADHD patients need lots of support as they deal with their problems and learn healthy habits. As with any disability, there are many challenges to support someone with it. Resentful or guilty of your partner's difficulties is not productive. It will only cause more stress in your relationship and increase the strain. Just being aware of what your partner is going through and making an effort to communicate with them is a great first step in balancing the relationship.

What You Can do

There are many small things that you can do to ease your relationship. You can balance out the tipped scales, and ensure that both parties are receiving what they need. Working together on these issues will increase your chances of success. Look for ways you can work together to meet each other's needs. You will be amazed at how quickly your relationship improves. These are some easy ways you can improve communication and ease some of your partner's stress.

* Your partner should stop talking and give your full attention to them. Ask your partner to focus on you and make sure they do not start talking to others. You will be able to stop them repeating themselves so often.

Listen to your partner and pay attention when they complain. If this is the case, then you should take steps to change your behavior. If your partner insists that you've been complaining about this same thing repeatedly but you don't remember it that way and you keep a diary, note the subjects and take steps to correct the behavior. When they bring up something, you can refer to them.

* If you believe your partner has forgotten something, apologize to them and make the task right away. You can ask your partner to remind you gently the first time, so that you don't become defensive and frustrated. This is something you work through together. You need to have the opportunity to improve your skills once you start using your new tools.

* If your partner suggests that you depart at a different time to the one you have proposed, then follow their lead. You might underestimate the time it takes for a task to be completed or travel to your destination. Let your partner lead the way if they are right.

* Avoid impulse spending. If this is a serious problem, it may be worth asking

your partner to manage your joint bank account and take over the finances. While you are improving your financial habits, there are other ways you can help to balance the work load and share responsibility.

* Keep a list with all your household chores. Aim to have a rotating system where you can swap turns, or designate who does what chores when it is convenient for you. To make sure you are both accountable to each other for household chores, write your name down on the list.

These are just a couple of things you can do for one another to strengthen your relationship. It is a good idea to meet with your partner, have an honest and open conversation about what's going on and discuss possible solutions. Don't accept blame for your partner's mistakes in the relationship. Relationships should be a team effort. Each person must own their mistakes and make efforts to help each other.

Adult ADHD can make it difficult to cope with. But you don't have the ability to do it all alone. Your partner should be supportive, loving and willing to help you achieve a functional and healthy lifestyle. If they are going to be able help you, then they need to know that you're open to them. Your partner should be invited to join you in the coping process. You both have much to give one another.

Chapter 13: Structuring And Organizing Your Daily Life

Living with ADHD can make each week difficult. It can be difficult to keep up with everyone else, feeling like you're always behind and not able to catch up. After a long week filled with running late, missing appointments and misplacing belongings, it can be refreshing to have a weekend off. Weekends are for catching-up, not resting.

Many fall prey to negative self-thoughts. "Why is this so hard for you to manage everything?" "I always fall behind." "I must be very bad at handling my life."

This type of self-talk is a stressor that makes it difficult to get through each day. Worse yet, it doesn't actually improve the situation. Even though you can be tough on yourself to the point of being blue in the face sometimes, the cycle will never change unless something is done.

The good news? These negative statements don't have to be true. One small step at time, you can put your life back in order. ADHD will require you to put in a lot of effort to get organized. However, once these structures are in place, you'll feel so much better. You can create these structures yourself, as many ADHD people have done it.

Get organized in your home

It's the place where your heart is and where you keep all your stuff. Our homes are our foundation. They give us a place for rest and relaxation, as well as a place for food, sleep, hygiene, and preparation for the day. The flow of our lives is directly affected how well we maintain our homes. A messy house means chaos, but a clean, well-organized home is conducive to a peaceful and orderly life.

It's much easier to know where everything is when you need it and you won't waste your time looking for it. It's easier to do what you love, which will help you get out the door in time.

Although it may seem daunting to organize your whole home, it is actually quite simple if you break it down and do each step one at a while. Here are some tips to help you make your home more conducive for living a life that flows.

You should always keep the same items in the same place. For important items like keys, coats and phones, keys and wallets as well as important paperwork, create a space. It's easier to remember where things are when you need them.

Break down the chores of cleaning into smaller, daily tasks. Take small steps each day when cleaning. This will keep the task from becoming overwhelming. Instead of putting dirty dishes in the sink, clean them up immediately if they are only a couple. Hang coats, hang dirty clothes, and place them in the hamper. It will help you live a more peaceful life and improve your focus and mood.

You can do whatever you want, as long as you have some spare time. It's worth taking a weekend to organize your house. You can use plastic storage bins and gallon freezer bags to organize your mess. Keep the most frequently used items close to your heart so you can quickly access them. It is important to label everything accurately so you don't forget about where you have stored them.

Do a deep clean at regular intervals. Make sure to schedule regular cleaning days to ensure that all the places you may not see in your daily life, such ceiling fans, lighting fixtures, or fine detail work in the kitchens and bathrooms, are cleaned up.

Structure your Daily Life

Your life will flow much more smoothly if there are clear plans and established routines. You will be able get to your destination on time every day with a solid structure, have everything you need for the day, and not let appointments or obligations slip by.

Routines, which are life structures that bring regularity to our lives, allow us to know what to look forward to every day. The ability to predict the day's events ahead of time allows us to have more control over what happens, how it happens, as well as when it happens. This level of empowerment will enable you to accomplish any task you set your mind.

It's important to take some time to ensure you are taking care of yourself. It's easy to forget the most important things in life when you're running late.

Get ready for every morning with a positive attitude. Preparing your outfits for the morning can save you time. Gather all the items that you will need for your day. These items should be located where you are most likely to see them as you go out the door. So you can remember to grab your stuff 15 minutes before leaving,

Use a routine to guide you through your morning. You must always follow the same order when completing your morning routine. These actions will become automatic and you'll spend less time rushing through your morning if there is a specific order for how to get ready, shower, style your hair, and brush your teeth.

It is important to know exactly how much time you will need to prepare for the day. You can time your morning routine for a week to find out how long it takes you for each step. You can then take the time that takes you the longest and incorporate it into your daily routine. If you find yourself frequently late, write down all the steps you have and see which can be combined with or eliminated. If you have to complete a task, such as eating breakfast in 20 minutes, then set a time limit and tell yourself that you will not be distracted by reading articles or running late.

You should keep important tasks at the forefront of your mind every day. Sticky notes should be kept where you can see them every day to remind you of important appointments, errands, or tasks. Keep them in a place you can see when you're done with the task and create new ones as needed.

Make sure you have enough food in your fridge and pantry. Keep a grocery list that you have easy access to. Add the item to your grocery list immediately you run out.

Plan to run errands at regular times. To go grocery shopping, pick a particular day of week. Set reminders and add the grocery shopping date to your calendar so you are always on track. If you have all you need for a successful week, your week will run smoothly. To complete other routine errands like dry cleaning or book return, you can set up similar processes. All your errands can be completed in one day.

Each person's life is different so no two will look the same. Our lives have many similarities so the same advice applies to all. You should consider your needs when you create routines and build your structure to ensure your life looks and works exactly as you desire.

Chapter 14: Daily Exercise And Adult Adhd

You all know how important exercise is for our health. Did you know that it can also benefit ADHD? Even though it might not be obvious, exercise is a great tool for managing ADHD symptoms. Recent research has revealed amazing results about the benefits of exercise for ADHD sufferers. Let's examine some of the many methods that exercise can help with adult ADHD symptoms.

Exercise has many benefits

Exercise has many obvious benefits, such as helping improve heart health or building endurance and strength. The brain also benefits from exercise. There is increasing evidence that daily exercise is beneficial, according to researchers. ADHD sufferers will benefit especially from the beneficial effects of exercise. Researchers have found that daily exercise can improve your health.

* It acts in the brain in the same manner as stimulants. The brain releases dopamine during exercise. Dopamine improves focus. Dopamine promotes consistency in the brain's attention system.

* Releases endorphins. These are hormone-like chemicals that regulate pain, pleasure and mood. Endorphins are what give you the rush of joy and energy after you get past the initial wall that blocks pain and discomfort.

* Helps to produce norepinephrine, which is a neurotransmitter linked to stress and focus. Daily exercise improves brain communication, boosts mood and releases the "happy chemical", serotonin.

* Has the exact same effects on the brain that Ritalin/Adderall. Although the effects

of exercise last for a few hours, it may not be enough to replace medications completely. Only you and/or your doctor can determine if exercise is a suitable substitute for medication.

* It improves executive functioning, which refers to the skills needed for planning, organizing, prioritizing, focusing, remembering details and a "working memory". Exercise improves inhibition (resisting distraction) as well as cognitive flexibility (the ability switch between tasks).

Chapter 15: Relaxing Or Unwinding

Adult ADHD is a challenging condition that makes it difficult for people to relax and unwind. The combination of anxiety and excess energy can cause your brain to run at 100 mph. This can lead to tightening up. It is important to relax and unwind in order for the body's energy to recharge and to get good rest. Your body will run on fumes if it is not given the opportunity to recharge. You can make your body more stressed than it needs to, and this creates a vicious cycle that is dangerous and unhealthy.

But, with dedication, you can teach your body how to relax. Relaxation can help you feel calmer and more relaxed, which will make it easier to reduce stress in your life. Here are some simple ways that you can relax and unwind every single day.

Stay present in the moment. Put aside all the things that have happened or need to be done to get to sleep. Put any unfinished tasks on a list and put them aside a few hours before you go to bed. After that, let yourself relax and enjoy the night.

Allow yourself to take breaks throughout the day. Your body will learn to relax by doing this. This can reduce stress and anxiety, which can prevent you from relaxing when they are high.

You don't have to relax to be healthy. It can be difficult, especially in countries like the United States, to have a positive attitude about rest and good health. Your work will improve if you have time to relax. You'll be more focused and less distracted throughout the day.

Incorporate relaxation time into daily life. You can get so busy that you forget about your body's fundamental need for rest. Just like any other task, you should also make time to relax and unwind every day.

You have a variety of options to help you unwind and relax.

* Yoga

* Getting massages

* Reading books

* Drinking herbal tea

* Take a slow, steady walk

* Hot bath

* Listening and enjoying soothing music

* Meditation

* Watching a soothing movie

Even though it takes some effort, you will see a big difference when you make the effort to take time for yourself every day. The effort it takes to train yourself to relax is well worth it.

Chapter 16: Time And Money Management Techniques

ADHD is a condition that makes money and time slip. It can be difficult to manage these two important aspects of life if you don't know how long things take or when due dates are. Everything else in life becomes chaotic when our time and money management is off track. These building blocks are essential for a successful life.

There are many tools and systems available to help you keep track how your time and money is being spent. To make sure you pay your bills on-time and complete your tasks on schedule, you can create systems that remind you. These systems can either be simple or complicated, but they are most effective when they are the simplest.

Time Management

It doesn't matter if you are late for appointments or meetings, or if you don't have enough time to complete tasks on time and meet deadlines. These time management strategies can help you stay on the right track and get more out of your time.

Use a planner. Planners are important for tracking tasks, appointments, and due dates. It is a good idea to keep your planner close by so you can quickly write down tasks or appointment as they occur. Make a habit of checking your calendar multiple times a days, every day. Even if everything seems clear in your head, double-check just to be certain.

Keep an eye out for the clock. ADHD patients swear that clocks should be placed in every room in their homes or offices. It is easy to lose time when you are focusing on a task. It is important to keep your eyes on the clock so you can stay focused and get the job done. You should place the clocks so that you can see the numbers at any location in the room. Take a note of when you start a project. Write it down or speak it aloud so that you can keep track of it. Timers can be used on your phone or computer to remind you when it is starting and when it will end.

Plan your week and month. As we learned in the chapter on productivity planning for the week, month, and weeks ahead will help you get a better understanding of what's happening in your life. You will be able to increase productivity and still have time to enjoy the things you love. Plan ahead and you won't forget anything.

Chapter 17: Healthy Living

We have seen the benefits of daily exercise for people living with ADHD. A healthy lifestyle goes beyond getting enough exercise. ADHD can only be managed if one is healthy in all aspects. Any one thing that is not in balance will affect the other. You will be able to manage your symptoms better and feel happier overall by adopting a holistic approach towards health and well-being.

Get lots of sleep

Sleep is the way the brain produces electricity to regulate all bodily functions. If you do not get sufficient sleep, your symptoms can worsen. Your symptoms will get worse if your brain has trouble producing these essential neurotransmitters.

One of the best things you can do to help your brain is to ensure that you are getting enough sleep every night. Regular sleep will help your brain focus better, avoid distractions, and retain information.

Keep Stress Low

Stress can disrupt the body's natural processes. High levels in stress hormones cause a rapid increase in heart rate, which can have a devastating effect on the body's organs. High stress can cause a variety of health issues later in life like heart disease, high blood Pressure, and many other problems.

Stress can also lead to more severe symptoms. Stress hormones in the body can cause your body to react faster and prevent rational thinking. In order to escape predators and save ourselves, we evolved this instinctive response. In modern times, this is often outdated, but long-term stress can cause us to remain in an inefficient state. Reduce stress will make your body and brain relax, and will reduce the severity of your symptoms.

Avoid Alcohol and Drugs

Many people with ADHD enjoy drinking and using drugs. ADHD sufferers often crave stimulation and novelty. Some people choose to self-medicate by using drugs or alcohol to help them relax. You should not gamble with your safety or health by using illegal substances or alcohol. These substances are highly addictive and can cause death.

ADHD sufferers will face many challenges, not only because of the obvious dangers but also because drugs and alcohol can pose a challenge. Alcohol and drugs can cause brain chemistry disruptions that disrupt production of essential compounds for memory and focus. You should avoid alcohol and drugs, as tempting as they might be.

Eat a Healthy Diet

The way you deal with ADHD symptoms can depend on how healthy your diet is. While a poor diet can lead to more symptoms, a good one can improve your ability to manage them.

A diet high in protein can increase your body's production neurotransmitters. They are essential for your ability to focus and remember, as we've learned in other chapters. Balanced eating with lots of fruits, vegetables proteins and whole grains will be a benefit to your body, while an unbalanced one will make you look bad.

ADHD sufferers need to eat foods rich in zinc, iron and B vitamins. Supplements that are high-in magnesium or omega-3s are also important. These minerals are crucial for the brain's production neurotransmitters like dopamine which are responsible to maintaining attention.

Avoid high-sugar foods and drinks. Sugar can lead to hyperactivity, leading to spikes and crashes in blood sugar levels. This can adversely affect concentration. Many studies have also shown that ADHD people are more susceptible to gluten sensitivity than those without it.

ADHD sufferers have access to a wealth of information on healthy living. It is important to consult your doctor before making any drastic lifestyle changes. But, with proper supervision and guidance, making steps towards a healthier lifestyle could have enormous implications on your ability to manage ADHD.